NURSING A PROBLEM

This book is to be returned on or
the last date s

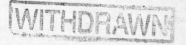

NURSING A PROBLEM

Lesley Mackay

OPEN UNIVERSITY PRESS
Milton Keynes · Philadelphia

610.73069094I MCK

Open University Press
12 Cofferidge Close
Stony Stratford
Milton Keynes MK11 1BY

and

242 Cherry Street
Philadelphia, PA 19106, USA

First published 1989

British Library Cataloguing in Publication Data

Mackay, Lesley
Nursing a problem
1. Great Britain. Nursing profession
I. Title
610.73′06′0941

ISBN 0-335-09902-5
ISBN 0-335-09901-7 (paper)

Library of Congress Cataloging-in-Publication number available

Typeset by Vision Typesetting, Manchester
Printed in Great Britain by J.W. Arrowsmith Limited, Bristol

Contents

Foreword   vi
Acknowledgements   viii

1   Introduction   1
2   Setting the Scene   4
3   Learning to be a Nurse   16
4   The System in which Nurses Operate   37
5   Constraints on the Job   55
6   Hopes and Aspirations: Discrepancies Between Nurses and Employers   73
7   Bitchiness   95
8   Who Looks After the Nurses?   113
9   Why Do They Do It?   132
10   The 'Good Nurse'   151
11   Change and More Change   158
12   Drawing the Threads Together   178

Appendices
1   Notes on the Research and Methodology   183
2   Previous Research: a Brief Overview   185
3   Questionnaire Sample Composition   186
4   Interview Sample Composition   187
5   Learners' Sample Composition   188
6   Number of Children   188
7   Number of Breaks from Nursing   189
8   Why Returned to Nursing   189
9   Doing Other's Work   190
10   Community Care   190
Bibliography   191

Foreword

Over the past year there has been quite unprecedented attention given to the situation of nurses both by the media and by politicians. Politicians were suddenly introduced to the problems of nursing without knowledge or interest in the subtleties of the issues; unions were seeking the common interests which bind their members together; and the media wanted a straightforward message which appealed to the sensibilities of their readers. For a while, politicians, unions and the media could briefly come together to confront the common enemy of low pay. For the rest, however, the picture is much more complex. Even among nurses, what are seen as issues for some nurses are not mentioned by others and vice versa. However, until we begin to understand the varying demands, interests and needs within the ranks of nurses, we may remain puzzled as to why nurses continue to leave.

Our starting-point for this study came at a time when the problems of the nursing profession were less public. Indeed, the study stemmed from our concern that, despite the fact that approaching half a million nurses are employed within the National Health Service, many issues surrounding nurse recruitment and nurse wastage had not been considered in a systematic way for many years. We have noted how the *Review Body for Nursing Staff, Midwives, Health Visitors and Professions Allied to Medicine* had commented in its second report in June 1985 that '*in the management's view* only a very small proportion [of nurses] left the NHS for reasons of dissatisfaction' (my emphasis). This was said at a time when some local health authorities were beginning to recognize they were experiencing some difficulties in the recruitment and retention of nurses. Clearly it was time to hear what *nurses* had to say.

Our concern has been to identify some of the recurring themes which emerge in conversation with nurses. We hope that these concerns are listened to, for otherwise they may remain recurring, but neglected themes. Certainly we continue to be amazed that in the heat of the intense debates about the future of nursing, few have tried to listen to what nurses have to say. This is a major attempt to fill this gap.

(Dr) Keith Soothill
Director, Nurse Recruitment and Wastage Project
Department of Sociology, University of Lancaster

Acknowledgements

The work on which this book is based was a team effort. I am most grateful and appreciative of the efforts by various members of the University of Lancaster for their contribution to the project. My thanks to Paul Bagguley, Jon Barry, Richard Davies, Brian Francis, Pisamai Kupituksa, and Moira Peelo.

The funding which made this project possible was gratefully received from the Leverhulme Trust. Similarly the cooperation and willingness of the Health Authority (which wishes to remain anonymous) to participate in the research was very much appreciated.

My own thanks must go to Keith Soothill for his unfailing support and encouragement throughout the project. In particular, my thanks go to all the nurses who spoke to me or completed questionnaires. I hope they like the book.

Lesley Mackay

1

Introduction

Nurses are a problem. They are a problem for their patients, for their managers and for their government. They also cause problems for themselves.

Nurses cause problems for their patients because there are often not enough nurses to go round. For managers in the Health Service the problem is that they are often hard pressed to keep the service going because of a shortage of nurses. Nurses present the government with another problem: nurses enjoy a great deal of public sympathy and support but they are not well paid. That is seen as the responsibility of the government. This demand for increases in nurses' pay puts further pressure on a government determined to limit the amount of public expenditure on the National Health Service. And nurses cause problems for themselves through their actions and attitudes to one another.

At the moment many nurses are voting with their feet and leaving the NHS, some never to return. In the recent past nurses have been treated as an easily replaceable workforce. This treatment needs urgently to be reconsidered because nurses may become an endangered species. The number of young people entering nursing is declining and the pool of suitably qualified, potential recruits is shrinking. This, by now well-known, demographic time bomb is being accompanied by a predicted increase in the number of elderly people.

We all need nurses at some time in our lives, especially as we become older and more frail. The demand for nurses will increase as the supply shrinks. Now is the time for policy makers and managers in the NHS to concentrate fully on recruiting and retaining as many nurses as possible. If worthwhile policies are to be framed then they will need to be informed by an awareness of the problems which nurses encounter and create as they work.

The main aim of this book is to focus attention on the experiences of nurses: their demands and their needs. Many of the demands of nurses for greater training, promotion and career prospects have fallen on deaf ears. Perhaps it is because most nurses are women. As women, they are seldom seen as such a valuable resource as men. Why else would the largest employer of women in Europe have so few childcare facilities or arrangements for flexible working? Received opinion about the way in which women and their careers are viewed has a large part to play in the way women are treated at work. Thus, women only play at jobs, merely waiting until they marry or have children and when they do return to work it is only for 'pin-money'. What a comforting view for men when jobs are in short supply. Such a view ensured that women at the end of the First and Second World Wars gave up their jobs, their careers and their recently found skills for the men who returned as heroes. It is a view, however, which is reaping a sad harvest in the NHS at the moment. Many women embark on a nursing career because they have a sense of vocation yet many of these nurses would not now choose to start nursing all over again. And most importantly, many nurses would not recommend the job to anyone else.

Nursing is a particularly stressful and demanding job. The stresses of the job are made worse by the reactions of nurses to one another. Many nurses speak of nursing as 'bitchy', where colleagues gossip and tell tales, picking on juniors and learners. Nurses often fail to give support to their colleagues and appear to have a lack of respect for each other and their particular skills. It is a mirror image of the way in which many members of the medical profession view nurses.

Doctors' interactions with nurses often leave a lot to be desired. A lack of respect, a wish for a 'handmaiden' together with a general condescension seems to epitomize the attitude of some doctors. Once again, the fact that most nurses are women appears to be highly influential. We all know there is little equality to be found in members of a health-care team. We all expect the doctor to be in charge, the nurse obediently and quietly doing his [*sic*] bidding. The relationship within the sphere of health care nicely reflects the domestic relation-ship. But, in both areas, women collude in defining the position to which they are allocated. This is not to deny the overwhelming influence of social, political, and economic factors in the way women see themselves. However, if nurses are to improve their situation they must take positive action themselves. The traditional resistance to 'political' action amongst nurses has engendered a tendency towards passivity and docility in other areas. But if nurses no longer wish to be 'kept in their place', and paid accordingly, this passivity must be abandoned.

The importance to nurses of a decent salary cannot be over-emphasized. Nurses are badly paid and they know it. Recent pay awards do little to bridge the gap between nurses and their peers in the police force. It is with the police force that nurses often compare themselves (quite a number of nurses either marry or have relatives who are in the police force). The disparities in pay between these two uniformed occupations are quite obviously due to the gender of the majority of their respective workforces.

Not surprisingly, gender is a recurring theme throughout the book. Gender fundamentally affects the way in which nurses are seen and see themselves. At the same time, nursing continues to be dominated by views which owe much to Florence Nightingale and the particular antagonisms of class and gender of a distant age. The fault, if there is one, lies with the nurses as much as with the system. There has been too little questioning of the accepted order within the ranks of nursing and the place of nurses within the hierarchy of health care.

The overwhelming dominance of the scientific view of health care is another theme which emerges frequently. Just as the way in which nurses are treated as employees will be questioned as nurses become more and more scarce, so the prevailing attitudes to health care will be questioned as health care becomes increasingly expensive.

Nursing is in the process of being changed. The many recommendations of the United Kingdom Central Council in *Project 2000* will undoubtedly have some impact on the experience of nurses and the development of nursing. Yet, as will be argued later, these 'external' changes need to be accompanied by fundamental changes within nursing – changes in the way nurses see themselves: as nurses, in relation to doctors and most importantly, as women.

The picture of nursing which emerges in this book is my view. However, I very much hope that it adequately reflects the views of all the nurses who have so kindly taken time to talk to me. Their co-operation has never been taken for granted. I am glad that many of the nurses found the chance to talk about nursing helped them. It is an indication of what is wrong in nursing today that these nurses often feel they do not have a friendly ear to turn to within the Service.

2

Setting the Scene

It is important to listen to what nurses have to say about their work. Nurses account for nearly half the workforce of the NHS and around one-quarter of all NHS expenditure is on nurses' salaries. Without nurses, wards are closed down, operations are cancelled, and casualty admissions directed elsewhere.

Nurses occupy a particularly interesting position in the provision of health care. Often they are the sole intermediary between the doctor and the patient. At the same time the nurse acts as the buffer between the patient and the potentially bureaucratic nature of the health service. Nurses are in the front line of health care. Listening to what nurses have to say acts as a useful barometer by which to measure the state of health of the NHS as a whole.

This book is based on interviews in one Health Authority with nurses who left and their colleagues who stayed, during the winter and spring of 1987. I have referred to these two groups as 'leavers' and 'stayers'. I also talked to two groups of learners at intervals throughout their first year of training. In addition I had conversations with some senior nurse managers. (For further information on the project and methodology see Appendix 1.)

Including all the occupations and work of these nurses under the one heading 'nurse' is misleading. For example, learners, both pupils and students, are trainee nurses: they are not yet nurses. There is an enormous variety in roles and skills of these nurses. There are Enrolled Nurses (EN) who train for 2 years as Pupils who have very limited prospects of promotion. In order to be appointed as a Senior Enrolled Nurse, enrolled nurses need to have a minimum of 3 years' full-time experience. The pay-scale of SENs corresponds to that of staff nurses. There are Registered Nurses (RGN) who train for 3 years as students. On qualifying, students become staff nurses. There are different specialities in which registered nurses can train such as mental illness, mental handicap, and children's nursing. Having worked as a staff nurse for a couple of years, further training in a specialty such as midwifery may be pursued. Midwives do not normally call themselves nurses. (A midwifery qualification is particularly helpful in achieving promotion and in moving into the community nursing services.) As an alternative a staff nurse may seek promotion to sister/charge nurse grade. Proceeding through the grades at sister level, registered nurses have the option of entering teaching or management. Clinical teachers teach in a practical setting while Tutors in the School of Nursing tend to be classroom-based. On the management side, promotion results by moving from sister/charge nurse level to nursing officer (or nurse manager as it is becoming called). From there, the Director of Nursing Services is the only hospital or service-based appointment. Thereafter, nurses move into general management and out of the clinical sphere altogether.

A questionnaire survey was carried out in the Health Authority (see Appendix 3). That survey gave some indication of fruitful lines of enquiry and of particular problems experienced by different groups of nurses. From time to time I make reference to this questionnaire survey as it also directed my attention to discrepancies between the accounts given by nurses in face-to-face contact with those formally given in writing.

The book's focus is on nurses' experience of work. The accounts that nurses give needs to be heard in their own words. It is the words that nurses use which most clearly reflects their view of their world. I have tried, as much as possible, to present nurses' accounts of their experiences in their own words. Had I used my own words more, and theirs less, the picture would be a less clear reflection of nurses' worlds. However, in choosing which parts of nurses' accounts to present in this book, the book reflects my own interpretation of their accounts. Although they are nurses' words, the choice as to what aspects to bring out is mine. My understanding of the way in which 'nursing' affected nurses developed as I talked to more and more nurses. Because I used a semi-structured approach to the interviews, I could pursue particular topics of interest to each nurse in greater depth. Had I used a structured approach with a fixed set of questions and asked in a given order, the result would have been akin to an elaborate questionnaire. My aim was to find out what nurses thought about their jobs and the aspects which they felt were important in their working lives. My 'theory' is embedded in the way I have written this book, in the questions I have asked the nurses and the way in which I have presented the answers. But it also results from listening to what nurses say and how they say it. As a result, I rely heavily on using nurses own words rather than superimposing yet another level of interpretation on their accounts.

I am not a nurse. I am an outsider looking in. There are obvious disadvantages in not understanding at first hand the particular demands and rewards of nursing. There are advantages in that as an outsider I am less likely to take for granted accepted working practices and attitudes. I hope, therefore, I can take an 'uncluttered' view of nursing. It seemed inappropriate at the outset to view nursing as an occupation similar, in broad outline, to any other. Nursing to me appeared to be 'special'. In particular, the apparently prevalent idea of 'having a vocation' is seldom found in other occupations. The occupation had, therefore, to be approached with caution.

As a result, the theory which emerges is 'grounded theory',[1] theory that is developed as the work progresses. I see little point in tacking on a bit of one theory here, another there, and thus ending up with a patchwork explanation of nurses' experiences of work. It was not obvious at the outset that the history of nursing, the gender of the workforce, the relationship between occupations, the relationship of nurses to one another, would each be extremely influential aspects of nurses' working lives. Had I started off with firmer 'theories', I should probably have reached different conclusions and pursued one avenue to the exclusion of others. Thus, the theory which emerges is also essentially a statement about the way in which sociological investigations ought to be carried out. Theories can act as artificial constraints on investigations. They can act as blinkers, directing attention to too narrow an area. Thus, the possibilities of explanation can become limited. This, of course, is not to deny that the development of a grounded theory has limitations. For example, it can focus too closely on present, and temporary, events or result in an ahistorical approach.[2]

Many books have been written on sociology and nursing, focusing on areas such as the organization of health care, the organization of nursing, professionalization, roles, and socialization. I am not going to rehearse all the arguments put forward in the realms of medical sociology. Aspects relating to these issues will be touched on throughout the book and reference made to other work which pursues further the ideas I have presented. The reader who is interested can consult a wide range of literature given in the bibliography. (For a brief résumé of some previous research relating to nurses see Appendix 2.)

Many of the problems facing nurses cannot be disentangled from the problems facing the Health Service. The Health Service is also sick. The NHS was described in 1979 as 'battered, bedraggled and worn at the edges'.[3] Its condition, 10 years later, is worsening. It may be going into a permanent decline. Government policies have focused on a number of areas which are fundamentally changing the face of health care in the UK. There are policies designed to increase the amount of health care provided by the private sector; to increase competition by the use of sub-contractors for various aspects of health services; to engender a more entrepreneurial spirit amongst NHS management; and, to make more efficient the use of resources which are given to the health services.

The knee-jerk reactions of 'leave the NHS alone' in response to attempts to alter the NHS are misplaced. The NHS may well have been a system of health care of which we could rightly be proud. Yet it is a gigantic organization which uses up a great deal of the national purse. Its organization and its aims need reappraising and redirecting. It is cumbersome and it has tended to grow without careful direction. It is not even clear that the health of the nation has improved as a result of the introduction of the NHS in 1948.

There is a health divide within Britain. Indeed, there are 'disturbingly wide' inequalities in health between classes.[4] The better-off enjoy better health than the poor. The better-off will live longer, and experience less sickness and ill health throughout their lives.[5] The way in which the NHS has been structured and perceived means that it is beyond its brief to address the underlying social problems of housing, unemployment, and associated deprivations which deeply affect health. Yet, 'a co-ordinated policy to reduce inequalities in health in the UK has not been adopted'.[6] The government has rejected the recommendations of the Black Report as being too costly. Instead the emphasis has been on making savings in the health budget, ensuring that value for money is obtained.

Undoubtedly there were, and probably still are, some economies which could fruitfully be made in the activities of the largest employing organization in Europe. However, some of these attempts have back-fired. Accounts of cancelled operations, lack of beds, and of unacceptably low standards of cleanliness, are increasing. Then there is the knock-on effect of all the economies on the nursing workforce. Many nurses are leaving, some never to return. It is not a loss which the NHS can tolerate.

Difficulties facing the NHS are not just confined to present or impending shortages of nurses. Questions need to be asked about the orientation of the NHS and wider issues surrounding health. The National Health Service has been called the National Illness Service.[7]

It is directed towards illness rather than towards health, and is curative rather than preventative in focus. It has been estimated that 5 per cent of NHS resources is spent on prevention, compared with 70 per cent on treatment and 25 per cent on caring.[8] Millions can be spent on treating illnesses such as heart disease, which, with education or social policies, can often be prevented.

Compared with other Western countries, the UK spends less on health care.[9] It has been estimated that in 1983 about 5.5 per cent of our Gross National Product was spent on health care compared with 10.5 per cent in the USA.[10] Yet, as regards our level of health, the UK 'surpasses several countries with much higher spending levels'.[11] The amount spent on administration is extremely small in comparison with our European or American counterparts. In the USA, 5.3 per cent of the health budget is devoted to the costs of administration, yet only 2.6 per cent is spent in the UK.[12] For the money we spend on health care, we receive good value. Undoubtedly, the NHS is still a system of which we could be proud.

The costs of health care, however, are rising. And our demands for health care appear to be increasing at the same time. Advances in medical science make more sophisticated (and often expensive) techniques available. We have come to accept that having a heart by-pass operation is a normal demand to make of the health service. While we make such demands of the acute sector within the NHS, others go without. Their demands for care are not being met.

The acute sector in health care enjoys a special position. 'The big spenders in the NHS are hospitals and they account for over 70 per cent of all NHS spending.'[13] The special position of the acute sector is maintained at the expense of others. According to the World Health Organization, there needs to be a change of perception towards 'a health system encompassing the total population rather than focusing on the limited groups such as hospitalized patients, self-referrals, and other ready utilizers of available services'.[14] At the moment, health care emphasizes 'the centrality of the curative process'.[15] For those for whom the notion of cure is inappropriate: the mentally handicapped, the physically disabled, the elderly and the dying, the NHS is less attentive. For example, the amount spent on food for mental patients is less than that for general patients.[16]

The distribution of nurses also reflects the primacy of the acute sector in health care. The largest proportion of nurses I talked to (47 per cent) are to be found within general hospitals with only 8 per cent working in the community and a meagre 1 per cent in the area of mental handicap (see Appendix 4 for details).

The proportion of NHS resources spent on caring is not high. Local government bears the brunt of responsibility for caring,[17] but the emphasis within the NHS is on curing. This reflects the dominance of the medical profession in health care. It is a dominance which is reflected in the press and the media where 'Health correspondents appear to be closer in orientation to their science-reporter colleagues than to social service correspondents.'[18] The dominance of the medical profession and the importance of 'curing' appears to be largely unquestioned by the general population[19] and by many nurses.

Thus, the system of health care we have in this country is in need of a substantial reappraisal. The ordering of priorities which favours acute care at the expense of the chronic; the favouring of a curative over a preventive approach; the inequalities in health between classes; are all aspects which need to be given careful consideration by those who allocate resources within the NHS.

Posing an additional problem in the NHS today are the number of nurses who are leaving. Nurses are fast becoming an endangered species. There are not enough nurses working in the NHS today. Shortages of nurses are being experienced in many parts of Britain, particularly in metropolitan areas, and especially in London.[20]

If enough recruits cannot be found and if nurses cannot be enticed to stay there are three possible outcomes: some nursing will be undertaken by less qualified personnel; some nursing will be undertaken by more highly qualified personnel; and, that less nursing care, and therefore less health care, will be available. Thus, without sufficient numbers of nurses, problems regarding the quality and quantity of health care are likely.

Nurses are leaving the NHS – a few to work abroad, some to work in the private sector, some leave nursing altogether and most because of domestic commitments. The numbers leaving the NHS has not been treated as 'a problem' until fairly recently. The need for changes in the way that nurses are perceived and treated has been apparent for years (see, for example, the findings of the Briggs Committee) yet action has been lacking.

In the past there has been an acceptance that the NHS can operate on a system of constant replacement of nurse learners.[21] That system no longer works. The number of young people entering nursing is declining. This is happening at a time when, due to demographic changes, the number of young people in the population is also declining.[22] Correspondingly, the number of young women (there are as yet few men in nursing) with five O levels is declining. Thus, the NHS needs to recruit an ever-growing proportion of school leavers if it is to keep the numbers of nurse learners at the present level.[23]

However, from recent research it appears that the number of schoolgirls who would consider nursing as a career is declining rapidly.[24] As a result there have been many calls to enlarge the scope of recruitment drives to include mature entrants, men, and those with good academic qualifications. At the same time, 'back-to-nursing' campaigns, to encourage ex-nurses to return, have been increasingly evident. Yet, many learners complete their nurse training but do not go on to register and practise as nurses. Thus, it is not sufficient to attract people to nursing, it is necessary to try to retain their commitment to nursing. Increasingly the government and managers within the NHS will have to focus their attention on keeping the nurses that they have already got. Instead of being treated as a disposable workforce, nurses will have to be treated as a valued and scarce resource. At the same time, greater attention will have to be paid to the demands and needs of nurses.

Leaving in itself is not necessarily a problem. In the 1970s there were fears that not enough nurses were leaving the NHS! Nurses can become stale unless they move into a different specialty or update their knowledge by undertaking further training. It is not always the best nurses who stay.[25] The high-fliers may be the ones who move on. When nurses leave, it is not just a simple matter of replacing them with others. When conditions of employment deteriorate and some nurses decide to leave, those who remain face increased pressures. If they were hard pressed before, the situation is made worse by every nurse who leaves. Thus, as the stresses and frustrations of nursing rise, morale will fall. A vicious circle is created.

Even if nurses do not leave, there are other expressions of dissatisfaction with work. Absenteeism can become a problem. In periods of high unemployment, as now, when the choice of alternative jobs is limited, nurses may simply not turn up for work. They may legitimately be ill or they may feel unable to take another day of pressure. Either way, the effect is the same: nurses who do turn up for work are put under even greater pressure than before.

At the same time, nurses under pressure may feel they have too little time to spend with patients. Conversations with patients can become brusque and impatient. The quality of patient care may suffer while nurses try to maintain the quantity. Two-hourly checks of temperature or blood pressure, for example, may still be carried out but patients may feel they are being treated as objects or that they are simply a nuisance. The perceived attractions of the private sector where the nurses can sit and talk with patients are made evident.

A full circle is completed where it becomes apparent that the pressures facing nurses are essentially linked to the pressures facing the NHS. By addressing the problems and the experiences of nurses, some of those pressures are more closely revealed. Many of the difficulties experienced by nurses result from political, social and economic changes rather than as a result of the characteristics of the workforce. Political influences reveal themselves through the initiatives of the present government on privatization; encouraging individual rather than national medical insurance; emphasizing 'community care' and individual self-help; strengthening the private sector and encouraging the competitive ethic. General social changes are apparent in the greater number of women in the workforce; in the feminist movement; in changing norms regarding childcare and mothers working (although the latter does appear to be under attack at the moment); and, in questions regarding the proper emphasis within the whole sphere of health care. On the economic front, the ever-increasing necessity for a family to have two incomes; the boom in consumerism; the reduced choice in alterative employment all combine with the political and social factors to provide a turbulent environment which an occupation and its members are currently facing.

However, account must also be taken of the composition of that occupation and how it affects the reaction to these pressures. That an overwhelming proportion (around 90 per cent) of nurses are women, with the majority being married and nearly half of them having children are important factors in the way these pressures are perceived. Many of the difficulties and stresses experienced by nurses are related to the fact that they are spouses and parents: problems of a partner getting, losing or moving jobs; problems of caring for babies, children, and teenagers. The impact of children on women's work-lives in particular can be dramatic. With children, balancing the demands of home and work can add a great deal of stress. The problems of home are brought to work and the problems of work are taken home. Extra responsibilities which come with promotion may not be welcomed. Part-time working may be the only way to cope. Yet the arrival of children means greater financial burdens and the need perhaps to work those hours which bring in the greatest income. The problems of young parents are particularly felt in nursing as it is dominated by younger people. Three-quarters of nurses are under 40 years old. Despite the relative youth of the nurses, many have substantial levels of experience. A large minority of nurses had over 10 years' experience in nursing, with a further third having 5–9 years' experience.

High levels of turnover amongst nurses are frequently reported in the media. Such figures need to be treated with great caution. Nearly half of the nurses who completed my questionnaire had one or more breaks in their nursing career. Leaving, in other words, is normal. Not only do nurses have breaks from their career, they move around a lot. At some time, two-thirds of the leavers (compared with just under half of the stayers) had moved within the NHS to do further training. Many moves are made by nurses to further their careers. Some nurses felt they had to move around in order to get the experience necessary for promotion. To some extent, moving around is an expected part of nursing in order to pursue one's career (such an expectation also exists within the medical profession).

To gain an appreciation of why nurses 'leave' it is interesting to consider the fifty leavers I spoke to. Of these, fourteen were leaving because they were pregnant or to look after their child/ren. Pregnancy is the most frequent reason given for leaving nursing (temporarily or permanently). There are particular problems for nurses as parents: early starts, late finishes, the weekends, the night duty, being on call, etc. The hours do not fit in with school hours or with the 'normal' hours of other occupations. The response of many nurses to these, perhaps temporary, complications is to go and work elsewhere. Many nurses return to jobs they have done before. They have worked in offices and shops, in factories, and in pubs. Apprentice joiners, fashion designers, computer programmers, teachers, and home helps come together in order to undertake training as a nurse. Around two-thirds of the nurses had worked in non-nursing jobs.

Fourteen of the leavers were moving to work elsewhere in the NHS and another five were going on to do further training. This latter move was normally made without any guarantee of a job at the end of the training. Four were leaving to take up non-NHS nursing jobs – in private nursing homes, in industry etc. Eight were leaving nursing altogether, one due to ill-health, one to failing her exams and the other six had some complaint about nursing. In total, a quarter of these 'leavers' were actually leaving nursing in the NHS. Contrary to popular stereotypes about great numbers of nurses leaving the UK to nurse in Saudi Arabia, the USA, or Australia, only one of the leavers was going abroad.

It is obvious that a high level of movement amongst nurses is both reasonable and predictable. Indeed, as mentioned earlier, there was concern in the late 1970s that it was not high enough![26] However, the constant movement of nurses has a number of 'knock-on' effects. When other nurses hear of yet another colleague leaving, for whatever reason, it affects morale. No one likes change and to have a constant movement of staff does not particularly help the smooth running of a ward or service. It makes the job of managers difficult in that they are constantly looking for replacements. The result may be that, in the short term, nurses are transferred temporarily, or that bank nurses are used. Again, this is unlikely to help morale. If temporary or permanent replacements for leavers are not found quickly, too few nurses have to do the work, causing stress and frustration amongst those who are left. In turn this leads to higher levels of absence. This, in itself, may result in a downward spiral causing more nurses to consider leaving. A high level of 'turnover' makes leaving seem normal while staying becomes associated with both a lack of career development and individual potential. Finally, a high turnover can result in divisions between 'old-timers' and the newcomers preventing any sense of camaraderie.[27] Of course, these causes and effects are not separate: they overlap and influence each other.

Recently, great stress has been placed on the potentially harmful effects of high turnover. However, greater recognition should be given to the normality of leaving. Movement within the NHS is not necessarily negative – it is good for nurses to broaden their experience. And nurses *can* become stale if they remain in the same specialty for many years. But movement is negative only if nurses themselves associate it with low morale or as a response to poor working conditions.

Despite a strong commitment to nursing, many nurses thought about other jobs they would like to do. On the bad days, there is an obvious pull to another job, sometimes *any* other job! Leaving seems to be a fairly frequent topic of conversation. Various constraints such as their own lack of qualifications or alternative jobs prevent some nurses from leaving. Serious consideration has obviously been given by quite a few nurses to leaving. Starting their own business was the most attractive option for the leavers I talked to. Further higher education was the most often mentioned choice of stayers. Some obviously felt they had made the wrong choice when they entered nursing.

More nurses should be leaving the NHS. As will be seen there is great dissatisfaction amongst nurses. But nurses tend to 'soldier on', comforting themselves with the idea that they have a vocation: they didn't come into the job for the money but simply to care for patients. If they were to leave, so some nurses argue, who then would look after the patients? The sense of responsibility given to nurses in their training ensures that the crisis within nursing will only slowly come to the surface as demographic changes take place.

Notes

1 Glaser, B.G. and Strauss, A.L. (1968) *The Discovery of Grounded Theory*, London, Weidenfeld and Nicolson.

2 Much has been written on the history of nursing, see, for example, Abel-Smith, B. (1960) *A History of the Nursing Profession*, London, Heinemann; Ehrenreich, B. and English, D. (1973) *Witches, Midwives and Nurses: A History of Women Healers*, New York, Feminist Press.

3 Garner, L. (1979) *The NHS: Your Money or Your Life*, Harmondsworth, Penguin, p. 172.

4 Whitehead, M. (1987) *The Health Divide: Inequalities in Health in the 1980s*, London, Health Education Council, p. i.

5 ibid. p. 14.

6 ibid. p. 93.

7 See Anderson, O. (1987) 'A national health service – in reality what can that mean?', *The Health Service Journal*, 29 January, 98:5035, p. 127.

8 See Harrison A. and Gretton, J. (1984) *Health Care UK 1984: an Economic, Social and Policy Audit*, London, Chartered Institute of Public Finance and Accountancy, p. 48.

9 ibid. p. 126.

10 ibid. p. 126.

11 ibid. p. 127.

12 Quoted by Garner (1979), p. 179.

13 Merrison, A. (1979) *Royal Commission on the National Health Service*, London, HMSO, Cmnd. 7615, p. 344.

14 World Health Organization (1974) *Community Health Nursing*, Geneva, WHO, Technical Report Series No. 558, p. 16.

15 Davidson, N. (1987) *A Question of Care: the Changing Face of the National Health Service*, London, Michael Joseph, p. 4.

16 This point is discussed by Tuckett, D. (1976) 'Doctors and Society', *in* Tuckett, D. (ed.) *An Introduction to Medical Sociology*, London, Tavistock, p. 380.

17 See Harrison and Gretton (1984), pp. 48–9.

18 Tuckett (1976), p. 272.

19 See Tuckett (1976), p. 392 who discusses the isolation of patients and their particular vulnerability to the mass media picture of medicine.

20 See Royal College of Nursing (1987) *Shortage of Nurses in London*, London, RCN.

21 United Kingdom Central Council (1986) *Project 2000*, p. 11.

22 See Dickson, N. (1987) 'Best foot forward', *Nursing Times*, 7 January, 831:1, p. 41.

23 See Bosanquet, N. and Gerard, K. (1985) *Nursing Manpower: Recent Trends and Policy Options*, University of York, Centre for Health Economics, Discussion Paper 9.

24 According to findings reported by Dickson (1987), p. 40, the percentage of schoolgirls who would *not* consider a career in nursing has increased from 61 per cent in 1982 to 71 per cent in 1985.

25 See Redfern, S.J. (1978) 'Absence and wastage in trained nurses: a selective review of the literature', *Journal of Advanced Nursing*, 3, p. 241.

26 See Redfern (1978), p. 231.
27 See Simpson, R.L. and Simpson, I.H. (1969) 'Women and bureaucracy in the semi-professions', *in* Etzioni, A. (ed.) *The Semi-Professions and Their Organization*, New York, Free Press, p. 245.

3

Learning to be a Nurse

For nurse learners the introduction into the system of health care is a crucial and extremely influential period. The received values and attitudes of nursing are passed down from the School of Nursing and its tutors to the learners. Qualified nurses working in hospitals and the community give further reinforcement to the traditions of nursing and the position of nurses. However, two different methods of nursing are learned at the same time: the 'proper' way and the 'realistic' way. Learners are isolated and abandoned to 'the system' when they step onto the wards. It is a traumatic time, a baptism by fire, which is visited on each new intake of learners and little attempt is made to soften the shock. The learners find a disheartened and debilitated Health Service which qualified staff battle daily to contain. The NHS seems unwilling to look after or care for its enthusiastic recruits to nursing. Is this because they are mainly women? Or is it because the system of nurse training needs to be carefully re-thought?

New recruits to nursing are often seen as 'initiates who have to be moulded into a system'.[1] It may be that the problems of wastage which have bedevilled nursing in the recent past can be traced back to this 'system'.

Recruits to nursing are in a position similar to that of apprentices.[2] For the most part they are meant to learn 'on the job'. Over 70 per cent of the 3 years which students spend in training is spent undertaking practical nursing. They do spend some time (approximately one-sixth) in the classroom in the School of Nursing. The remainder is taken up by holidays. Learners account for 20 per cent of the workforce involved in nursing.[3] The Royal College of Nursing estimates that three-quarters of nursing care in hospitals is given by learners.[4] Thus, learners have an extremely important contribution to make to the delivery of nursing care. It is by no means obvious that the importance of this role is recognized by those who train and supervise the work of these learners.

Although the learners are meant to be training, they are included in the numbers of staff allocated to a shift on a ward: they are *not* supernumerary. They are expected to learn as they work[5] and they have to work hard. Thus, learners, instead of being trained, are often treated as just another pair of hands.[6] Like many apprentices, the training they get often results from 'sitting next to Nellie'. Poor practices and short-cuts are often the basis of the learning on the wards. It is in the School of Nursing, away from the hustle and bustle that the unreal, but correct, way of working is learned. Learners have 'to come to terms with two versions of nursing'.[7] Seldom is time available for training sessions in a clinical setting. Greater importance is given to the demands of the 'service' than to the learners' needs for training. Having to meet the immediate and increasing demands made upon them, the permanent staff make use of all the people they can. The pressures are too great to allow learners the space in which to learn properly. The suggestion in the UKCC's *Project 2000*[8] that learners *should* be supernumerary is timely.

At the moment, however, learners are not supernumerary. They have to put their heads down and work. As they work, doing (initially at least) the more basic nursing duties, they learn what is expected of them: from patients, from staff, from tutors. On each allocation – to a ward or unit – they learn what behaviour is rewarded and what is frowned upon. Learners learn about the system in which they are working. It is a peculiarly closed system for the possible introduction of new ideas. Nurses are taught by nurses. Thus, a 'perpetuation of practice without evaluation' and 'a treadmill effect' can result.[9]

As they go through their 'Cook's tour' they can see for themselves the different approaches and expectations in the different units. But there is little contact with disciplines outside nursing. Changes taking place in other areas of activity do not have a great chance of being heard let alone being influential. As a result the received knowledge within the ranks of nursing remains fairly static. It is not surprising, therefore, that nurses are often seen as conservative and reluctant to change. There is a tendency to keep looking backwards to the role model of Florence Nightingale. It could be argued that the light from her lamp shines too brightly, eclipsing the future potential and development of nursing and nurses. This may be especially true for the system of nurse training, which as Bradshaw reminds us, is now into its second century.[10] How does this century-old system work? Two groups of recruits to general nursing were followed through their first year of training. Contact with both groups of learners was made in their first week in the School of Nursing. Their help was enlisted – all volunteered to participate – in the project which had been given the go-ahead by the staff in the School of Nursing.

The learners came from a wide range of backgrounds. Some came straight from school. Others had taken time out to obtain the O and A levels necessary for acceptance into nurse training. Only one had not worked before. Five pupils and three students had experience in jobs which were allied to nursing such as care assistant or auxiliary. Experience in shop or office work was also common (6 pupils and 7 student learners respectively mentioned these). Four learners, and they were all pupil nurses, had worked in factories. Only student nurses had worked in technician-type jobs. Seven learners had worked in pubs or as waitresses.[11] Many of these jobs were temporary stop-gaps while they obtained further qualifications or waited for admission to the School of Nursing. Some work was voluntary, and some was part time. Other learners had worked for a few years in full-time permanent jobs. Experience of other work gives a benchmark against which nursing can be compared.

In choosing to do nurse training, by no means all recruits had wanted to be a nurse since childhood. Just under half of the students and pupils said they had wanted to nurse ever since they were children. While a third decided to take up nursing when they were in their mid-teens, nearly one-fifth of the learners did not decide until they were in their late teens. The older learners only decided to take up nursing in the 6 months or a year before they actually started their training. It is interesting that a third of these learners had not decided what they wanted to do by the time they left school.

For many of these learners taking up nursing meant doing further O and A levels. While they were taking further qualifications they had plenty of time to reconsider their decision to go into nursing. Three-quarters of the learners who were followed through their first year in nursing had taken some further training after leaving school. Not all but most of this training was taken with nursing in mind. There appears, therefore, to have been quite a strong commitment to a nursing career amongst these learners which survived the time spent preparing to enter nursing.

People enter nursing with their own stereotypes as to what awaits them. Many of the stereotypes are 'filled out' by relatives and friends who are nurses. Only two learners had neither a friend nor a relative who was a nurse. It appears that consideration of nursing as a career is often associated with the presence of someone fairly close at hand who has experience of nursing. Thirteen of the nineteen learners who knew a nurse had been encouraged to take up nursing. The apparent salience of these recommendations should be borne in mind by those who seek recruits to nursing. Nevertheless, such encouragement frequently included warnings about particular aspects of nursing. One-third of the learners mentioned 'hard work' as the main warning they had received. The delights of bedpans had also figured prominently but only in the warnings remembered by students. Perhaps because bedpans are an expected part of the enrolled nurse's duties there is little future in them objecting to them! For students on the other hand, bedpans are something they can effectively rise above once qualified. Thus a distaste for bedpans can be expressed in the sure knowledge that they are not a long-term hazard.

The need for dedication, in order to do the job well, was mentioned by pupils and students. 'Dedication' is linked to a notion of vocation which is ever-present in discussions about nursing. Thus it is believed that nurses are born and not made. However, only two learners mentioned this aspect. This suggests that the notion of vocation is weak amongst recruits and that it is instilled during training. As the learners come into contact with demanding and trying situations their ability to 'take it' may be linked to the depth of their vocation for nursing. In other words, if you can't take it, you do not have a vocation for nursing. And if you can take it, you have obviously got a vocation.

The learners enter nursing with fears: of being unable to cope in emergencies, squeamishness in dealing with large wounds, of giving their first injection, of coping with death and the dying and being alone on a ward at night. These are common fears amonst recruits to nursing.[12]

While learners' friends and relatives primarily warned about the content of the job, the learners worried about how they, as individuals, would cope. (NB All names are pseudonyms.)

> . . . we were all really frightened the first day.
> . . . you think you're going to get thrown in at the deep end when you're not really. But you feel as though someone's going to ask you to do something . . . (Kay)

Not all the learners were apprehensive. Some entered with confidence, having had experience in looking after patients in other settings before. A quarter of the learners had formed no preconceptions. Their attitude was of the 'I don't know until I've tried it' variety.

The point is worth emphasizing: only one-quarter of the recruits came into nursing with an open mind, without particular fears. Three-quarters of the learners had specific or general fears about their ability to cope with situations or meet the demands put on them.

Learners' early prejudices regarding particular wards or specialties are not often borne out. Learners, in being given their 'Cook's tour' of the various specialties, find attractions and disappointments every-where. For example, twelve of the twenty-one learners mentioned paediatrics as the specialty they felt they would most like. Yet by the end of their first year only a few pupils who had been given experience in paediatrics expressed a preference for it (students are allocated to paediatrics in their second year).

After a few weeks in school the learners move onto the wards. Their first ward is often tiring. Indeed, the hard work and their tiredness are recurring themes in their conversations. 'When you get off a late it's often too late to go out and you are often pretty tired. Some days I get so tired I just go to bed.' (Paula)

At the same time the learners have to adjust to the shift system. The shifts seldom follow a predictable pattern and it is difficult to plan any social event if it is more than a couple of weeks away. Special occasions, say 2 months hence, mean that learners have to make contact with the sister/charge nurse on their next allocation in order to try to get the day off.

The ways in which shifts are patterned is compounded by having to work 10 days in a row. These '10-day stretches' as they are called (in language remarkably similar to a prison sentence) on duty with no days off are universally disliked by these learners. 'I think these 10-day stretches should be abolished – they are terrible. We've all had them. You're absolutely shattered.' (Sally)

Then there are the weekends. Learners often seem to draw the short straw when it comes to weekends off. Some pupils complained about having had only one weekend off in 8 or 9 weeks.[13] While this may suit parents with younger families who have a partner at home, single nurses may have to substantially readjust their social lives. In time they adjust to the shift system of earlies and lates, coming off duty at 9 p.m. and going back on duty at 7 a.m. the next morning. But further adjustments are needed. Having become used to one shift pattern they then have to become used to another. For example, the students are given experience in a psychiatric hospital where they operate a 12-hour shift. The shift pattern was predictable and that was appreciated, but for some students the shift was simply too long. The shift systems offer particular problems to nurses with younger families. They do not coincide with either school hours or normal working hours. It appears that learners are often unfairly treated with regard to shifts and weekends off.[14] Certainly, the learners often *felt* unfairly treated in this respect.

Learners also have to learn to cope with the responsibilities and the pressures of being unsure and facing strange situations. 'Sometimes I feel like a fish out of water. I feel very alien. There is still a lot I have to find out about. I feel a nuisance sometimes . . . (Dorothy)

While in the School of Nursing the learners were often impressed by the scope and responsibility of the work they would be doing. The work was normally a good deal more responsible and involved a greater degree of autonomy than they had experienced before. They worried as to whether they had the ability to meet the demands which they felt were going to be made of them. And they worried that they would be just a 'spare part': an encumbrance rather than a help to the trained staff. To feel part of the team was much prized.

> I like feeling useful really, that I can do something. When you're at [nursing] school it's just sort of sitting around, listening and learning and you think 'God, I'll never be able to do this' but when you get there, once you've done it once then it's alright, it's just . . . feeling you're part of a team – you're joining in. I really like it! (Yvonne)

The fear of exclusion was to emerge again and again throughout the different ward allocations. It was felt particularly strongly in those specialties which were self-contained or geographically isolated. But exclusion was also felt in wards undergoing changes and where staff morale was low. Learners appeared to act as scapegoats for the frustrations of the permanent staff. Because the learners were only 'passing through' there was less need for permanent staff to 'get on with them'.

> There was one girl who used to pick on me all the time – she was just a cow. [An enrolled nurse] and she used to be very sarcastic: sarcastic comments coming out left, right and centre every day. I got really upset . . . (Clare)

In being seen simply as passing through or as a pair of hands, learners as individuals with their own fears and problems are ignored.[15]

The attitudes of permanent staff are critical. If the permanent staff are not supportive and aware of the insecurities of the learners, life can be miserable. For most learners, however, the staff on the first ward allocation were reported to be kind, helpful and approachable. There was obviously relief in getting on with the permanent staff.

> They're [the staff] really nice – they really looked after me. As soon as I went on they put me with somebody for the first few days and they looked after me. (Kay)

Where the staff are not approachable, when the learner is being told off all the time and no appreciation is given, then the learner thinks about leaving.[16] When the learners go onto their second ward allocation they have to face a completely new set of circumstances: new staff, different medical conditions, new routines, different practices, and different attitudes to learners. It is a traumatic time, they have managed to build up some level of confidence after their 8 weeks on one ward but most of this confidence vanishes the moment they step onto a new ward.

> You just get used to it, then you are moved on. (Sally)

> Part of me is looking forward to it but part is apprehensive because I don't know what is expected of me. (Wendy)

> I get really worked up and anxious when I go onto a new ward because you don't know what to expect at all. We were shown round the ward on Friday and they really just didn't want to know – they just showed us round the ward and then we went, and they seemed really awful. (Kay)

But the first week on the new ward passes and the learners settle down again. They know they are outsiders and this makes all the more keen their desire to be treated and perceived as 'part of the team'. The experiences of learners in this respect vary tremendously:

> The other students on the ward and pupils, they're very friendly, but the permanent staff – they seem to let you know that you're not a permanent member of staff. It's a bit of 'us and them'. (Susan)

> . . . in the morning you were lucky if you got a 'good morning' off one of the staff. (Molly)

> . . . they made me part of the team right from the start. And the more I felt I could do, the more they let me do. They weren't sort of following me around all the time. (Yvonne)

The learners have by now got over many of their initial apprehensions: of giving their first injection, of seeing their first dead person and 'laying them out'. These early experiences are trying. Tears are often shed as they encounter some of the harder facts of life and of nursing. The unexpected death of a patient, the shock of being assaulted by a patient, witnessing the mistreatment of patients by trained staff are some of the difficult moments of nursing mentioned by the learners. They have become used to being called 'nurse'. In the beginning this often felt strange, but by now they have grown into the role – they are no longer acting.[17] Although they become accustomed to working as a nurse, the relationship with the other staff remains critical throughout their first-year allocations. Whether the staff are 'good' or 'bad' substantially affects the learners' experiences of nursing.

On a few wards the lack of empathy with learners of some permanent staff was evident. Some nurses had obviously forgotten how clumsy and uncertain learners can feel.

> The charge nurse was quite rude to the students and made you really lack confidence because he used to criticize everything you did even if it was right. (Molly)

> Sometimes I get a bit upset when somebody asks you to do something and you don't know how to do it, so if you do it a bit slower or ask, sometimes they're a bit impatient – I don't know whether they do it for your own good, sort of make you learn it quicker – but that sort of upsets me sometimes. (Heather)

Other nurses seemed to enjoy underlining the status differences within nursing. 'Some of the staff are very nice here but there are a lot who are a bit aloof, you can't really get to know them, especially if you're a pupil nurse (Wendy). It was obvious that difficulties with permanent staff increased the amount of strain experienced by learners . . . sometimes I come home and cry, but that's only on the odd occasion. I just want somebody to listen really; a bit of pampering, a bit of attention' (Ann). Giving care every day to patients, these learners would obviously like to receive some care themselves.[18] The learners know they work hard but they seem to receive little praise. When praise is given, it stands out above all else, knowing that their contribution is valued. For one student the best moment in 8 months of nursing was when:

> One morning, me and my friend were working the same bays and it was just us two looking after those two bays. And this EN, a new EN, told us that sister had said that we had worked well, very efficient – and it made my day. She [the EN] wasn't supposed to tell us that. (Molly)

It seems as though praise is felt to be bad for learners. The lack of encouragement to learners has been noted before.[19] Withholding praise and positive feedback from learners may lead them, once they qualify, to behave in the same way. A critical environment is perpetuated and the amount of stress felt by nurses and learners increased unnecessarily.

Only a few learners did not find nursing stressful but for most the stress came from a lack of knowledge or experience, insufficient support from staff, or the pressure of work itself.

> The pressures of trained staff sometimes on students. They expect them to know much more than they actually do. And just the stress of having patients' lives in your hands, working with people that are very poorly – you worry about them when you go home and get involved – you're not supposed to, but you do. (Theresa)

Some learners find it easier to maintain a distance from their work than others:

> I just don't think about it. I do definitely try and cut myself off from it – definitely. You can't come off the ward and constantly think about all the awful things and all the poor people that are on there otherwise you'd be in a right mess. (Alice)

It is not always an event which has already happened which is experienced as stressful. It may be the fear of the unexpected, the emergency, not knowing if she can cope:

> I can't pin it [the stress] down to anything specific. It's just sort of a feeling when I'm on the ward – you never quite know what's going to happen . . . (Heather)

The stresses of nursing for learners have been described elsewhere.[20] Learners face pressure because of the nature of the job and because they are learners. Many of the pressures of nursing appear to come from understaffing. All the learners mentioned understaffing as being a critical factor in many allocations. General surgical and medical wards seemed to fare worst. The understaffing had direct and immediate spin-offs in that trained staff had little time to spend with learners.

> Staff shortages mean you don't have anyone to supervise you if you are doing anything wrong or not. You don't know – you are just thinking 'am I doing it right' and there's no one to guide you. (Peter)

It alters the type of nursing experience which learners obtain.

> . . . you don't have enough time on the wards, not for the sort of thing that I think is important which is sitting down and talking to people. You don't get time to talk. (Heather)

It can mean that learners are given too much responsibility. In fact two-thirds of my learners felt they had been given too much responsibility at some time.

> On the ward you are given a lot of responsibility but its up to you whether you take it. I mean you can always turn round and say 'no I don't feel confident at doing that'. But usually it's just shortage of staff, it's a question of you've got to really. (Yvonne)

It can be frightening: 'Sometimes there are only three or four on. If something goes wrong and someone arrests, I think I wouldn't know what to do' (Paula). And finally, there is little time to spend with the patients. Patient contact is one of the most important practical aspects of nurse training. All the learners felt they had too little time to spend with patients. Learners often felt guilty if they were seen talking to a patient:

> There was times when I felt really guilty just sitting down and talking to somebody when there was so much to do – they obviously needed somebody to talk to. I found that really hard. (Ann)

> Because of staff shortages, if the staff see you sitting talking to a patient they will always come up and tell you to do something, whereas they don't really think that talking to a patient is doing anything – skiving the work really. (Julie)

Understaffing goes a long way towards making bad nurses. That is, nurses to whom the patient is an encumbrance, getting in the way of the work that the nurses have to get through on their shift. The negative effects of understaffing emerge starkly from the learners' accounts. The learners have not yet learned to take low-staffing levels for granted. And they do not take the lack of time with patients for granted. The understaffing was both shocking and disheartening.

Not having enough time with and for the patients was a continual complaint from the learners:

> No there's not enough time. I think that is what a lot of the patients need is to have a chat. One stroke patient just screamed the other day and when I went over and asked if she was in pain, she said no, she was lonely. She just wanted attention. I talk to her, she gets a bit confused – but they do need to have chats with people. Some of them hardly get any visitors, their families don't come in much. (Dorothy)

> . . . when you do have the time to sit and talk to them they start to cry because they wanted someone to talk to ages ago. (Sheila)

Working, as Dingwall puts it, is 'doing things'.[21] It is caring for the physical rather than the psychological and emotional needs of patients. If nurses are not doing something physical they are not seen to be working.[22] In this view, the role of a nurse becomes exceedingly limited. Patients are increasingly seen only as patients who have something specifically wrong with them rather than as people who are going through a period of ill-health or who are in need of care. Patients become objects. The increasingly short stays in hospital and the use of 5-day wards combine to reduce the quality of nurses' contact with patients.

The importance of patient contact for the learners should not be underrated. The aspect which learners like best about nursing is contact with the patients. Helping, talking, joking, and just looking after the patients is THE raison d'être of learner nurses. Learners need to feel appreciated by the patients, to be thanked, to be remembered and to feel valued by them. There is a great deal of dissatisfaction with the lack of patient contact. Such dissatisfaction has both immediate and longer-term implications. Immediate, in that learners don't enjoy the job as much when one of their main sources of feedback is denied them. The longer-term implication is that nursing, as it is experienced on a day-to-day basis, does not meet these learners' needs. They then leave nursing for a more rewarding job. At the same time they would not recommend anyone else to start nursing. Thus, nursing receives an increasing amount of bad publicity.

Understaffing was an influential factor in the discrepancy between the School of Nursing and actually working on the wards which some learners reported.

> You get a shock when you come into the wards – a great shock.
> In school they said that everybody will tell you how to do it. But
> you are thrown in at the deep end. I don't think the training quite
> prepares you . . . (Alice)

There are also the discrepancies between theory and practice.

> Training helps – it gives you an idea of what to expect, but
> putting it into practice is different. A task that takes half an hour
> in theory takes 10 minutes in practice on the ward. (Dorothy)

At one level such a discrepancy between the 'proper' way and the 'realistic' way is predictable. 'Going by the book' is not always possible. However, the discrepancy between theory and practice may be increasing as staffing levels are 'tightened'.

> . . . the way they do it in School is always long-winded and
> when you are on the ward there are a lot of short-cuts you have

to take. Being in School makes you aware of how things should be done whereas on the wards I don't think they're always done as they should be. (Kay)

Only a small part of learners' time is spent studying. While on the wards, learners are assigned a clinical teacher who is responsible for ensuring that the learners have properly covered some of the basic aspects of nursing such as doing a drug round, setting up oxygen tents, etc. Relations with the clinical teachers are not always good. Learners often complained of some clinical teachers' failure to visit them regularly.[23] It was obvious that a couple of clinical teachers were more assiduous than their colleagues. At the same time, clinical teachers' social skills were not always apparent.

. . . she said I wasn't assertive enough. She tells you off in front of the patients. She doesn't tell you off on your own. I feel you lose face a bit. I'd rather she did it on a one-to-one basis. (Sally)

Being told off in front of the patients was a complaint only heard from the pupils, not one student mentioned this happening. It does suggest that there may be different standards (as well as different types) of instruction given to the two grades of nurses.

I asked the students and pupils if they felt pupils were treated differently from students. Half the students felt pupils received less teaching on the wards. 'I think perhaps they teach the students more, and they show more interest because they know that you have more exams and a lot more bookwork' (Kay). Some students had remembered particular incidents in which pupils were denigrated by staff and student nurses. Corroboration that such incidents had taken place came from the pupils.

On children's ward two students had said to one of the other girls 'where's the playroom?' and she'd shown them and they'd said: 'Oh, how degrading having to ask a pupil where the play area is'. (Katy)

The pupils clearly felt a difference in status. Most pupils reported particular difficulties with students.

I think we're all looked down on by student nurses. (Sally)

Qualified staff have been really good as far as I am concerned towards pupil nurses. It is students that you have all the problems with. They'll come out with statements like: 'This is how WE make a bed' . . . they treat you as if you know absolutely nothing. (Alice)

However, the differences in treatment of students and pupils can be exaggerated. Two or three incidents were recounted again and again by the learners. It is possible that some pupils' lack of confidence and insecurity caused them to pounce on these incidents. But, whether imagined or real, divisions are perceived to exist between the two levels of nurses by most learners. It would be surprising if the perception of differences was not carried throughout their nursing careers.

All learners felt they had been taught most by staff nurses but enrolled nurses and learners further on in their training also played a part.

> It's the third-year students – they know what I need to gain experience in. And some of the newly qualified staff nurses are good as well. But I find that ones that have been there for a couple of years get very out of touch with what students need. (Heather)

> I think at first it was a staff nurse, a male staff nurse, the first few days but then really it is more the enrolled nurses I think . . . you can go to all of them if you're stuck on anything. (Kay)

However, there was fairly broad agreement that ward staff did not have enough time to teach learners.

> Not really no, a lot of people say 'if we had the time we'd do this' . . . (Theresa)

> On my ward at the beginning there wasn't any training at all really because the ward next door to us had just shut down and we were so busy I was just an extra pair of hands at the best, so I didn't get any training really. But since the ward re-opened they have been paying a bit more attention to me. (Heather)

> . . . there's times I've been asking staff nurse something in the sluice or something and sister will come along and walk past and even the staff nurse has felt guilty because she's explaining something. She's sort of hurried it and carried on with her own work. (Alice)

Lack of time for trained staff to teach learners is compounded by the need for learners to push themselves forward in order to be taught. Time and again the learners said they had to ask in order to find out: self-help training really. Such a method of training is not very suitable for the more reticent. 'You had to go and ask and if you didn't you wouldn't get taught. It's not so good if you're one of these people who stands back' (Ann).

For many of the learners, training on the wards was a hit-and-miss

affair. If a ward was well staffed, if the permanent staff were willing
and prepared to teach, if the learner was not afraid to speak up and ask
questions, and if the clinical teacher visited the ward regularly, then a
reasonable amount of training would take place. However, the ideal
was not often encountered.

Sixteen of the twenty-one learners felt they were not given enough
feedback about their progress and performance on the wards. Indeed,
comments on performance were usually made when the learners
were given their final ward report, and too late to make
improvements.

> They seem to tell you when it is too late. I think they should tell
> you as you go along and not wait for your interview to tell you. I
> would like to know as soon as I am going wrong. (Patricia)

Comments were often too general, e.g. 'you've done very well'; 'you
could do a bit better'. The need for detailed and frequent feedback was
apparent:

> I like encouragement. I like being told I'm doing alright to keep
> me up because I think 'what do they think of me? am I doing this
> right? am I doing it wrong? should I be doing more? am I
> overdoing it?' and things like that. (Laura)

The system of giving interim and final reports on ward performance
does not meet the day-to-day insecurities and worries of learners.
They wanted to become good nurses and to do a good job. Not
knowing whether they are doing well or badly militates against the
development of their self-confidence. At the same time, the unwillingness to praise learners adds fuel to the belief that nurses do not look
after one another.

Further difficulties with training face learners. They are expected to
undertake some studying and exam preparation while on their ward
allocations. Obviously there are problems in trying to work and study
at the same time.

> It's coming up to the exams. You feel too tired to study and guilty
> when you don't study. I think we all feel the same – we'll be glad
> to get back to School for the rest, after the exams! (Sally)

> Studying gets on top of you – it really gets on top of you. The last
> thing you want to do is pick up a book after a day's nursing.
> (Wendy)

While such great emphasis is placed on practical work it is often
difficult for learners to develop confidence regarding their essay-
writing or exams. Learners continually referred to their poor exam

technique, the particular problems of multi-choice questions and
writing essays:

> . . . my problem is the essays. I'm not brilliant at putting down –
> I tend to know it but not be able to put it down like they want to
> hear it. (Sally)

> The only thing that worries me is not doing so well in the
> exams . . . It's just the writing – I've got to practise getting all the
> information down in a legible form within the time. (Yvonne)

Given the importance of theoretical input to nurse training, the
present system fails to maximize the learning potential of these
nurses. The practice of trying to squeeze exam and essay preparation
into the working day is likely to be counter-productive. Tired people
do not readily absorb information. They are unlikely to perform well
in examinations. It would be only too easy to make hasty judgements
on the academic potential of these nurses which would not be to their
advantage. Cramming studying in with so much practical work may
also be counter-productive. Studying becomes an activity done under
pressure and rushed. Learning is unlikely to be perceived as a
potentially pleasurable pursuit. The present system is a perfect way of
ensuring that nurses do not seek to further increase their knowledge
once they have managed to qualify.

It is surprising therefore, as will be seen later, that many qualified
nurses do express great interest in doing further nurse training.
Nevertheless, the conditions for learning for new recruits in nursing
are less than optimal and the sooner they are changed the better.[24]

Given the limited opportunites facing the pupil nurses once they
qualify, I asked whether they would consider doing a conversion
course and becoming registered nurses. Over the year the views of the
pupils changed. For many, initial interest had waned by the middle of
their first year. The difficulties of combining studying and working
may have had some influence. Of course the additional demands and
responsibilities placed on staff nurses become more apparent as pupils
progress. 'One minute I want to, the next I don't think I do when I see
the staff nurses with all the hassles . . .' (Sheila). However, at the end
of 12 months this pupil said she was definitely going to try to get on a
conversion course. The report on *Project 2000* came out during these
learners' first year of training. The Report's plans to phase out the
enrolled nurse grade obviously put increased pressure on the pupils to
consider converting.

Many of the pupils were uncertain if they could handle the
responsibilities which they saw staff nurses taking. They mentioned
their own lack of confidence, their fear of taking responsibility and

coping with the many pressures on staff nurses. Yet these pupils did not differ so greatly from the students in their paper qualifications. Most of the pupils felt they would be able to obtain further O and A levels and to successfully complete the conversion course. What seemed to be at issue was their lack of confidence. Boosting of self-confidence was not overly apparent in the course of nurse training. Praise was seldom given. When praise was received, it was very highly valued. Learners, it seems, 'are never summoned for praise to be given'.[25]

As the pupils progressed through their first year they somehow gained in confidence. And it was towards the end of the year that some pupils commented that they felt wrongly advised to do enrolled nurse training. 'They did not mention student training at all. I think they should have said 'why don't you wait and . . .' – they should have advised us anyway' (Patricia). There was an implicit rebuke to the senior nurses in the School of Nursing to the effect that they should have been able to recognize pupils' ability at the initial interview. A few of the pupils felt unable to or didn't want to take on the additional responsibilities of the staff nurse grade. But it was clear that some of the pupils felt they had the ability to undertake student training. Whether or not any of these pupils would have returned to college to obtain the requisite number of O and A levels is another matter. They did, however, feel that the different options open to them within nursing could have been more carefully explained at their initial interviews for nurse training.

At the end of their first year the learners were asked if nursing was as they imagined it to be. Seven learners felt that broadly speaking, nursing had met their expectations. Six learners, all students, felt nursing was harder and more tiring than they had anticipated.

> . . . on the wards you are just running up and down all day doing this and that and the other and you are on a late and the next morning you are absolutely shattered when you get in and the next morning you are on an early. I hate that, it's awful, but it's got to be done though. (Susan)

Three pupils felt that nursing was more skilled and required greater knowledge than they had expected. Two students also mentioned this aspect, commenting further on the amount of responsibility they had to bear. Slight disappointment was registered by four pupils. Nursing was not as glamorous as one had thought. Another found nurses quite bitchy, while the hours and the staffing levels were mentioned by two other pupils.

As mentioned earlier, the most liked aspect of nursing is contact with the patients, yet lack of patient contact was a recurring complaint. When the learners were asked what was the aspect they least liked about nursing, they tended to focus on particular tasks. Bedpans, doing 'observations', back-rounds, the smells, giving out teas, were some of the tasks mentioned. These tasks were disliked because they were now seen as boring. The initial enthusiasm for basic nursing slowly wears off as learners' skills and experience develop. By the end of their first year many of the learners appeared to want more 'exciting' tasks. At the same time, however, there is often some disdain from the learners for staff nurses' wish to be 'in the office'.

All the learners I talked to felt they had been changed by becoming a nurse. Most comments related to what might be called 'personal growth'. An increase in confidence was mentioned most often by learners while becoming more understanding and better listeners was also frequently mentioned. Quite a few students and pupils felt more mature and said they had grown up in the year or felt they had become less shy. For the other learners there were different changes: of becoming more emotional, more moody. Four students and one pupil felt that they had become harder.

> You become a bit more hard. Yes, if people die it doesn't affect you so much. A man had his leg chopped off the other day and it didn't affect me at all. I always thought I would be so sympathetic and that it would get to me but it didn't bother me at all. (Clare)

The shell which some learners felt they had grown was by no means watertight. Particular incidents stood out and some patients could not be forgotten. 'The educational value of much clinical experience can be compared to exposure to ultra-violet light. Some get badly burned, a few are healthily brown and some get in the shade at the earliest opportunity and come away untouched.'[26] Two-thirds of the learners said they would still choose nursing again. However, the disparities between preconceptions and reality were substantial enough for a third of the recruits to think they would, if given the choice, opt for a different career.

Half the learners had considered leaving at some stage in their first year. One-third of the learners had considered joining the police. At first glance it seems a curious alternative choice. However, both occupations involve a great deal of contact with the public, have to cope with emergencies, are uniformed and command some respect in the community at large. The main attraction of the police was the pay. Pay is a source of great dissatisfaction for learners.

Most learners, if they were considering another job, would choose to work in some caring occupation such as social work or working as an auxiliary. By the end of 9 months in training most of the learners were firmly committed to completing their nurse training. Thus there were comments such as 'I couldn't do anything else now' and 'There's nothing else I want to do.'

Of the eight learners who would not choose nursing again, two were simply going to complete their nurse training and then look for another sort of job. Others mentioned the lack of other alternative employment or felt that as they had already completed a fair bit of their training, it would be a pity to waste it. Similarly the qualification enabled nurses to travel: ' . . . what's 3 years out of your life? It's nothing and it's qualifications which can take you anywhere so you might as well stick it out' (Ann).

Over three-quarters of the learners said they would continue to nurse after they qualified, but not necessarily in the NHS. Seven mentioned they would like to do nursing overseas, sometimes with the Army (one way in which an enrolled nurse can work as a nurse abroad). Whether or not any learners will actually go abroad is another matter (only one leaver was going abroad to nurse). Travelling abroad appears to be a topic often discussed amongst nurses and maybe given greater importance than it warrants as a reflection of nurses' actual career choices. Similarly, only two learners thought they would actually apply to join the police force.

The nursing aspirations of the students were greater than those of the pupils. This is hardly surprising given that there are few further training opportunities for enrolled nurses. Amongst students, midwifery was a popular choice for further training and slightly less frequently chosen, working in the community.

Many of the learners' plans after qualifying involved moving on – inside the NHS and outside it. Some students had entered nursing because the qualification would enable them to travel and work abroad. By the end of their first year, these learners have become used to moving about. Nursing was not seen as work in which you stayed in one place for any length of time. This is hardly surprising, given that as learners they are constantly on the move. They become 'tourists'.[27] Whatever the ward or specialty, whether a good or a bad one – it doesn't last for long. With this knowledge the learners can console themselves when they are not enjoying an allocation. The hope that the next allocation will be a 'good' ward makes negative experiences more bearable. It has been argued that constantly moving around as learners makes the settling-down phase after qualifying more difficult.[28] The current methods of training, in other words, may only make worse the movement that exists within the

NHS as well as the amount of 'wastage'. At the same time, it may be that once qualified, if staff keep moving and don't stay long enough in any specialty they fail to sufficiently develop their own nursing skills and potential.

This system ensures that learners receive little idea of stability or belonging. They are 'passing through' and in each allocation the aim is to obtain a good final report. The reliance of learners on the goodwill of permanent staff means that learners have to 'behave' themselves. Learners who speak out, ask too many or inappropriate questions, may be labelled as cheeky or as troublemakers. Not surprisingly, learners learn to keep their mouths shut and to do what they are told to do. It needs to be remembered that almost all members of staff on a ward can tell a learner what to do. The learners learn to take orders and to see themselves at the bottom of the pile. They are also discouraged from thinking for themselves and questioning accepted practices. They even learn not to speak out too loudly about bad practices as well.

It was exceedingly difficult for some of the learners to come to terms with poor nursing practices. None of the incidents related to me could in any way be attributed to understaffing, workload or stress. The 'winding up' of mental patients, just to 'get a rise out of them' could find no easy excuse. They were incidents which caused the learners a great deal of distress and they also felt helpless. To do anything about it, to complain, ensures the label 'troublemaker' follows them through from one allocation to the next. The dumping of a suitcase on top of a recently dead patient by a qualified member of staff was an incident which was extremely distressing to one learner. In such cases, learners may remonstrate with the culprit, or talk to another member of staff, but to officially report a trained member of staff was baulked at. (At least one attempt by a learner to initiate discussion of such an incident in the School of Nursing was sidestepped.)[29] About half-a-dozen separate incidents were reported where the behaviour of a qualified nurse left a great deal to be desired. For the learners to come across such behaviour is bad enough. To have to keep their mouths shut about such incidents demoralizes because in keeping quiet, the learners feel they are 'going along with it' – and that is *not* how they want nursing to be.

The learners feel isolated when they embark on their nursing careers, they want to be accepted and part of the team. Yet because they do have to 'bite their tongues' they know they only partially fit in. As a result, they are likely to learn to distrust other nurses who appear to fit in only too well. It is not surprising that in such an environment, learners come to accept, like qualified nurses, that nursing is bitchy. By accommodating themselves to the hierarchical system[30] and denying themselves as individuals, the frustrations of nurses can be expressed through bitching about colleagues. The way in which learners are treated ensures the continuation of this extremely self-destructive behaviour amongst nurses. With greater support, sympathy and understanding for the situation of learners a positive environment for change and innovation within nursing could be created.

Through all the stages of their training, students and pupils breathe the same air as trained nursing staff. They take on board the same, or at least similar, attitudes as those held by their more senior colleagues. This socialization ensures the continuation of nursing and its ideologies without challenge. Lacking the input from other disciplines into nurse training or while learners are receiving training, a narrow, introverted world can be maintained.

The constant movement of learners, the lack of training received on the wards, the poor support given to learners by qualified staff and tutors, the pressures of simultaneously studying and working, the isolation and failure to build up confidence in the learners – all point to an inadequate system of training. It seems as though the energy and enthusiasm of these learners has been abused. This abuse is not simply the result of the way in which the training is constructed – although the system does not seem to actually help. It is also the result of the pressures which the trained staff are facing along with everyone else in the health service. It would be surprising indeed if nurse training could be in a healthy condition when the rest of the NHS is not. But, in failing to meet many of the needs of nurse learners, management in the NHS does itself a disservice in that it fails to ensure the continued commitment of its workforce.

Notes

1 DHSS (1972), p. 70.
2 Whittaker, E. and Olesen, V. (1978) 'The faces of Florence Nightingale: functions of the heroine legend in an occupational sub-culture'. *in* Dingwall, R. and McIntosh, J. (eds) *Readings in the Sociology of Nursing*, Edinburgh, Churchill Livingstone, p. 27.
3 Qualified staff account for 56 per cent and 24 per cent are auxiliaries/assistants – Royal College of Nursing (1986), *A Manifesto for Nursing and Health*, London, RCN, p. 4.
4 Royal College of Nursing (1986) p. 6.
5 This 'dual role' is discussed in MacGuire, J. (1969) *Threshold to Nursing*, London, Bell, p. 9.
6 This evaluation of the position of learners has been voiced elsewhere, see RCN (1986), p. 6; Reid, N.G. (1983) *Nurse Training in the Clinical Area – Volume 1: The Report*, The New University of Ulster, p. 5.

7 Melia, K. (1984) 'Student nurses' construction of occupational socialisation', *Sociology of Health and Illness*, 6:2, p. 138.
8 UKCC (1986).
9 See M.O. Clark (1984) *in* Duncan, A. and McLachlan, G. (eds) *Hospital Medicine and Nursing in the 1980s: Interaction Between the Professions of Medicine and Nursing*, London, Nuffield Provincial Hospitals Trust, p. 49. The isolation of nurse learners from broader fields of education was also noted by UKCC (1986), p. 10.
10 Bradshaw, P. (1986) 'Think before we link', *Nursing Times*, 9 April, p. 51.
11 An association between nurses and manual work has been made by Clarke 'Getting through the work' *in* Dingwall and McIntosh (1978) p. 75. With regard to her sample of nurses in a psychiatric hospital such an association was less evident in these recruits than in general nursing.
12 See Birch (1975) p. 54.
13 DHSS (1972), p. 13, also found dissatisfaction amongst learners regarding weekends off.
14 See Clark, J. (1975) *Time Out? A Study of Absenteeism Among Nurses*, London, Royal College of Nursing, p. 45 and DHSS (1972), p. 71 respectively.
15 Salvage, J. (1985) *The Politics of Nursing*, London, Heinemann, p. 71.
16 See also Firth, H., McIntyre, J., McKeown, P. and Britton, P. (1986) 'Interpersonal support amongst nurses', *Journal of Advanced Nursing*, 11:3, pp. 273–82.
17 Bond, J. and Bond, S. (1980) 'Sociology: in touch with reality', *Nursing Mirror*, 28 February, 150:9, p. 27.
18 This point has also been made by Menzies, I. (1970) *The Functioning of Social Systems as a Defence Against Anxiety*, London, Tavistock, p. 33 and Stewart, B. (1981) 'In need of tender loving care', *Nursing Mirror*, 12 March, p. 35.
19 Lombardi, T. (1987) 'Under control', *Senior Nurse*, 6:5, p. 8; Johnson, M. (1986) 'A message for the teacher', *Nursing Times*, 31 December, 82:52, p. 42.
20 See Birch (1975).
21 Dingwall (1978) *in* Dingwall and McIntosh, p. 80.
22 James, N. (1984) 'A postscript to nursing' *in* Bell, C. and Roberts, H. (eds) *Social Researching: Politics, Problems, Practice*, London, RKP, p. 131.
23 Other researchers have also found that learners do not often see clinical tutors, e.g. Reid (1983), op. cit., p. 82.
24 See the recommendations of the UKCC op. cit. (1986).
25 Johnson (1986), op. cit. p. 42.
26 Bradshaw (1984), op. cit. p. 11.
27 See Pape, R. (1978), 'Touristry: a type of occupational mobility; *in* Dingwall and McIntosh op. cit., p. 56.
28 See Melia (1984), op. cit., p. 148.
29 For a discussion about 'collusion' in keeping malpractices quiet, see Tuckett (1976) 'The organisation of health care: a crucial view of the 1974 reorganisation of the National Health Service', *in* Tuckett op. cit., p. 249.
30 Others have commented on the way in which nurses are taught to be obedient and submissive to authority: Lombardi (1987), op cit., p. 8; Whittaker and Olesen (1978), *in* Dingwall and McIntosh, op. cit., p. 29.

4

The System in which
Nurses Operate

The relationship between nurse and doctor is marred by failures to communicate and cooperate, at least from the perspective of nurses. Doctors are frequently reported by nurses to be rude and condescending. Nurses would like to be treated with greater respect. Gender as well as class differences obviously have a role to play here. Responsibility for the troubled relationship lies not only with the attitudes of some members of the medical profession but also with the system of nurse training in which outdated attitudes to the medical profession are perpetuated. While training, learners learn their place, not to speak until spoken to and not to offer opinions. Nurses' silence ensures the dominance of the medical profession. However, the attitudes of nurses themselves do little to improve the situation. The anti-academic school of thought in nursing seems to enjoy some popularity. Thus nurses argue the need for practical rather than academic skills. Similarly the benefits of discipline are extolled. Although the nurse's role is currently being extended, for example, through the nursing process, it appears that the feminist movement is only tentatively reaching the ranks of nursing. Even now, it appears that the employment conditions of nurses are being further eroded.

The learners learn to survive in a system of nurse training which is both old and resistant to change. Qualified nurses also face a system. It is a system both conservative and hierarchical in which the medical profession dominates. The relationship between doctors and nurses is one aspect of this system which critically affects the experience of nurses. The relationship is fraught with difficulties and failures to communicate. The fact that most nurses are women and most men are doctors is relevant. Issues of gender appear to be inseparable from

issues which relate to divisions in skill and expertise between doctors
and nurses. However, not all nurses are women. Ten per cent of the
nurses I talked to were men. In order not to confuse issues when
looking at the relationships between doctors and nurses it is necessary
to consider what, if any, differences exist between women and men
who nurse.

It might be thought that male nurses would differ from their
colleagues in their views on nursing. However, on almost every topic
male nurses' views were indistinguishable from those of their female
colleagues. Despite commonly held assumptions amongst female
nurses that men find nursing pay particularly low, there was no
evidence that men were more concerned with pay than women.
There was no evidence that men were more or less militant than
women in nursing. It appears that an orientation towards nursing or
the socialization that takes place within nursing overcomes differences which might be encountered between the sexes in other
occupations.

How do their colleagues see male nurses? Many more men are to be
found in the specialties of mental illness and mental handicap.[1] But
the presence of men in nursing generally seems to be taken for
granted. *Male* nurses were never mentioned without prompting,
except to remark that nurses' pay was insufficient for men with
families.

I asked twenty-six nurses (including two men) if male nurses were
as good as female nurses. Half of them said men made as good nurses
as women. Nearly all the rest felt male nurses were more career
minded and tended to aim for 'glamorous' areas of health care. Nearly
a quarter thought men were not as good as, and/or lazier than,
women. The need for male nurses to be chaperoned when with female
patients was occasionally mentioned as it presents difficulties when
staffing levels are low.

Only a small minority felt discrimination in favour of men took
place. Thus, it was argued, more men reached senior positions in
nursing. There *is* a disproportionate number of men in the higher
grades of nursing.[2] Whether there is actually discrimination in favour
of men is open to debate. It has been argued, for example, that once
men achieve senior positions they tend to promote one another.[3] It is
the case, however, that according to the questionnaire data, men
have significantly fewer breaks in their nursing career when compared with women. It has been found elsewhere that men (who are
members of the RCN) do not work as part-time nurses.[4] The lack of
career breaks and the fact that men nurse full time means that their
road to promotion is much smoother.[5] 'While men are being

promoted or gaining experience that will equip them for promotion, many women are at home tending babies, their skills growing rusty and their knowledge lagging behind new developments in their fields.'[6] Even if women do return to work while they have young families, there are barriers to promotion if they only work part time. Despite men tending to come from a lower social class and to be less educated, they do achieve a disproportionate amount of promotion in nursing.[7,8] I asked these twenty-six nurses why they thought most nurses were women. One-third of them felt it was because traditionally nurses were women. A quarter said it was due to gender stereotyping so that men didn't even consider nursing as a career. In other words, as the husband of a sister was told, 'nursing is not a man's job'. The others felt men were less suited to, or interested in, nursing.

It doesn't appeal to men really – cleaning up after people . . . (Enrolled Nurse)

Most of the men I know would not be able to cope with blood, incontinence, diarrhoea – they would be sick and rush off to the toilet. (Enrolled Nurse)

The level of nurses' pay was thought by just a few to be not enough for a man. 'I don't think a male nurse could support a family on the wages we are on. The wages are disgusting' (Enrolled Nurse). Just a few said that the patients wouldn't accept male nurses but nearly one-fifth maintained that more men were now coming into nursing. (There is, however, little evidence to support this.)[9] The main reason given for men entering nursing was a lack of alternative employment when local factories closed down. It is not clear that this is actually the case. From the questionnaire data, nearly half of the men, who were nursing in the Health Authority, were 35 years old or over compared with just over a third of the women. This suggests the influence of factory, and other, closures on the numbers recruited into nursing took place some years earlier if, in fact, this did occur. Interestingly, one nurse pointed out that nearly half the nurses in the Army were men. (Five of the nurses had trained to be a nurse in the Armed Forces.)[10] It seems that the stereotyping of nursing as a women's job is confined to the civilian sphere and the specialties other than mental illness and mental handicap.

Overall, there appear to be few differences between the men and women who nurse. However, it has been suggested that the relationship between male nurses and doctors might differ from that between female nurses and doctors.[11] Only one charge nurse mentioned this aspect and his comment had to be qualified. 'They listen to me but less to women. It is a cultural thing. They [the doctors] are all Asian or Burmese' (Charge Nurse). No other male nurses mentioned any difference between themselves or their female colleagues in their relationship with doctors.

Wright also suggested that the relationship between female doctors and nurses may be different from that with male doctors.[12] The student nurses were asked if there was any difference in the way that female and male doctors treated nurses. The great majority said that women doctors and consultants tended to treat nurses rather better than their male colleagues.

> All the female doctors that I've met have been great, especially one of the doctors on medical, she was doing a liver biopsy and she explained everything to me. She explained absolutely everything she was doing and why she was doing it. It was really interesting, whereas I think a male doctor would just have gone ahead and said right I'm doing this, that and the other and gone ahead and done it and not explained exactly what they were doing. (Clare)

> They are all different. I suppose on the whole female doctors are more approachable, they are perhaps easier to work with, but there are exceptions. (Heather)

There are fewer female doctors than male and students' opinions appeared to be drawn from one or two experiences with female doctors. Nevertheless, most students did feel that women doctors were easier to work with than males. Women were held to be 'less arrogant', 'more helpful', 'nicer', etc. It is not clear whether the 'better' relationship with female doctors was due to the nurses' perceptions of women or because of the different behaviour of female doctors compared with their colleagues. There may be no difference in the way that female and male doctors see nurses. It has been suggested, for example, that women in the medical profession have taken on board, like their male colleagues, a scientific ethos of health care as distinct from the humanitarian qualities associated with nursing.[13,14] Given that women doctors are felt to be nicer than men, what sort of relationship generally exists between doctors and nurses? The label 'doctor' covers a wide range of medical personnel. There are junior and senior house officers, registrars, consultants, and general practitioners. Some members of the medical profession, such as anaesthetists, are often referred to as a breed apart. (For the sake of simplicity, I shall use the term 'doctor' to encompass all the different members of the medical profession – it is obviously a great over-simplification.) Similarly, the diversity amongst these 'doctors' in level of skill, age, and ethnic origin ought to be remembered.

Similarly, the seniority of nurses will affect their perception of, and relationship to, doctors. The age, grade, and experience of the nurse will also be influential. 'Oh I don't have anything to do with them at all – I'm the bedpan queen! I'll show you where the sluice is!' (Student). About a quarter of the nurses I talked to felt the relationship between themselves and doctors/consultants to be good.

> Because it's a specialized unit and you've got to get to know your staff and to be able to depend on what they tell you . . . There don't seem to be any problems. (Staff Nurse)

> They are very friendly and very nice. In casualty it is a bit different, we work with each other a lot more than you do on the wards. (Enrolled Nurse)

It was frequently pointed out that relationships tended to be better in specialist units or units that were geographically separate. The degree to which doctors and nurses are familiar with one another's working practices is likely to affect relationships.[15] Styles of working and the amount of contact also varied between specialties. For example, doctors are less often seen on long-stay psychiatric or geriatric wards. And nurses working with the mentally handicapped may well have virtually no contact with doctors. In such areas, there is greater demand for the skills of nurses than of doctors. As a result, doctors have a less interventionist role and their presence is less critical than, say, in a surgical ward. In such a situation nurses appear to develop greater confidence in their own abilities and there seems to be less deference to the medical profession. 'Its very different in psychiatry. You are very much the doctor's handmaiden in General' (Student). Nurses working in the community enjoy quite a degree of autonomy and this affects the way in which they relate to doctors.

> I've never had any quarrel with either of them. They're both pretty reasonable. They have to be persuaded. Neither of them are particularly difficult. If I want either of them to go and see somebody, they will go, immediately. (District Nurse)

In some areas of health care such as midwifery, relationships with doctors can be particularly difficult where areas of doctors' and nurses' expertise overlap. Challenges to the position or omniscience of doctors are an important factor here. A number of doctors seem reluctant to admit that nurses' knowledge, in some areas at least, could be greater than theirs.[16] Or, that, for example, nurses can take a much more prominent role in preventive health care.[17] Highly skilled nurses are less likely to be subservient towards doctors. In areas of health care where nurses enjoy considerable autonomy, such as in the community or midwifery, there is potentially a greater chance of friction between doctors and nurses. In midwifery, for example, not only are midwives highly trained but they help train doctors.

> The consultants are very good. The SHOs [senior house officers] that come – a lot of them haven't done obstetrics since their student days so when they first arrive they don't really know what they're supposed to be doing – they have a general idea obviously, but basically you have to teach them . . . Then after a week, two weeks, the SHOs are then telling you what to do which is a bit . . . [laugh] – that can get to you after a while. (Staff Nurse)

A quarter of the nurses I spoke to felt unable to make any generalizations about the relationship between nurses and doctors because of the variations between doctors in behaviour.

> We have doctors who lord it over us, you know 'get me this, get me that'. Then you have the other type who are very good. The eye doctors are all very good with patients. I think we judge the doctors by how they treat the patients really. (Enrolled Nurse)

Over a third of the nurses reported that relationships with doctors were not good. Complaints about the 'invisibility' of nurses were made, especially by enrolled nurses and learners.

> I don't like them too much. I mean I'm sent to get patients' notes and they are in the doctors' coffee room. I went in and asked, you know, where's such and such notes and they just ignored me and I saw them on the table in front of them. (Molly)
>
> One of my first days on the scrub side in theatre, one of the consultants just came up to me and sort of moved me out of the way like a piece of furniture. He didn't acknowledge I was there or anything at all. He just sort of moved me along and I was just totally dumbfounded. I couldn't believe it – I just stood there. (Ann)

Learners' views are of particular interest because they highlight aspects of doctors' behaviour which qualified staff may take for granted. The learners have increasing contact with doctors as they progress through their training. Doctors do have a role in teaching nurses: showing learners what they are doing and why they are doing it. Obviously some doctors enjoy this role more than others.

> The consultants would sort of shout at some of the qualified staff like 'why isn't this done?' but they didn't say anything to the pupils. They were really quite helpful. Like if they had the 'scopes out and things like that they'd say 'come and have a look at this nurse' and they were alright with the pupils . . . (Katy)

Of course, having learners asking questions and hanging on every word of wisdom can be a gratifying, ego-building exercise for doctors.[18]

While learners are given information on treatment and diagnosis by doctors they become accustomed to the way doctors work. They come to accept that doctors can shout, be rude, condescending, or obnoxious. The learners may have to accept doctors' behaviour but they certainly don't like it. I asked the learners how they felt doctors *ought* to treat nurses. The resounding reply was that nurses should be treated with more civility and respect.

> . . . treat you as another person, not just the scum of the earth or something. (Alice)

> Well I think they should treat nurses with respect. I mean we treat doctors with respect. Alright, maybe they've more qualifications than we have but they couldn't do their job if we weren't doing our job properly. They couldn't because we're sort of running the ward when they aren't there and they're only coming there for a percentage of the time. (Katy)

Sometimes the learners have been shocked by the way trained nurses respond to doctors.

> I was told when I was down in theatre that once, one of the surgeons had forgotten his own clogs so he put some wellingtons on and the sister went out of the theatre because he was in such a bad mood and she hunted high and low for his clogs. She came back with his clogs and she crawled under the table and put them on for him. And I thought is it any wonder that nurses are looked down on by doctors, if the sister will do that? You know, crawl under the table and put his clogs on just to cheer him up. Really, its hardly surprising is it? (Clare)

Such colourful incidents were only occasionally reported. (They

may take place often but no one notices or comments on them!)
Nevertheless, there is a continuing assumption amongst nurses that
doctors can and will behave badly. A doctor is valued because he or
she is not rude or arrogant.

> The doctors are alright here – they are not the sort you've got to
> be quiet on the ward round or anything like that. (Enrolled
> Nurse)

> I think you've got to have a personality and perhaps be a little
> cheeky and argue if you don't think something's right. Now that
> doesn't go down well. I have been in that position twice, where I
> haven't agreed with what's been done. But who am I to say? . . .
> They can make life difficult if they want to. (Sister)

> . . . in some situations you've got to stand up for yourself a little
> bit more than others, but on the whole, everything is fine. The
> consultants, they have set routines and we know to honour
> those routines, and we are quite happy and the patients do very
> well under them, so . . . (Staff Nurse)

> One doctor, I think she's very rude, her manner leaves very much
> to be desired – I feel she tries to belittle you. You know, for minor
> things that aren't really that important, she'll make you feel very
> small in front of junior staff about it. You know 'why aren't these
> X-rays here?' and that sort of thing. (Sister)

Doctors are obviously responsible for their own standards of behaviour. Although doctors' attitudes and behaviour will be much
influenced by their socialization during their training, they still have a
choice as to how they behave towards nurses. Nevertheless, some
nurses pointed out that part of the blame for doctors' behaviour rested
with nurses themselves and the way nurses were trained.

> I feel that I was always taught to look up at doctors . . . and I find
> it hard to get out of it really. (Enrolled Nurse)

> you are taught to respect them in the sense of fearing them and I
> think that's wrong. I don't think you should have to go to work
> and be frightened of anybody. (Staff Nurse)

The way in which nurses relate to doctors is part of an ethos which is
passed on to new recruits. Nurses, in essence, have to learn to know
their place.

> . . . you're trained to be submissive really. You're trained not to
> bark! Not to make a noise, to do everything quietly. I don't think
> there is enough assertiveness training in the actual training . . .

> It's because it's a very hierarchical system and the hierarchy tend
> to pass it down all the time. (Staff Nurse)

Senior nurses are certainly aware of the way in which doctors often
behave. Their comments corroborated the statements made by other
nurses. And the senior nurses voiced their opinions of doctors in just
as strong terms as other nurses.

Some senior nurses, however, felt that the attitudes of nurses to
doctors generally was in the process of changing and being changed:

> Now we question [doctors] and I encourage people to question
> much more than they used to. I think that the girls that are
> entering now when they are ward sisters, yes, there *will* be a
> difference, but I think not at the moment. The medical profession
> definitely think they are one up on them. (Nursing Officer)

In some places doctors can 'get away with' poor behaviour to
nurses whereas in others they cannot. An important factor is the
attitude of the sister towards her nurses and doctors:

> I've got some sisters who can stand up to the doctors and stand
> by their nurses. It depends on the sisters. If the sisters are
> prepared to do everything and say 'yes' to everything the doctor
> wants then the doctor will do it and get away with it. But if the
> staff are prepared to say you are not right and they question
> them, then the doctors are not quite as bolshy as they might be.
> (Nursing Officer)

It has been noted elsewhere that if a sister is not always present on a
ward round then over-confident young doctors may well get away
with more dictatorial behaviour towards nurses.[19]

The attitudes of nurses towards doctors may be changing (see
below). The learners were more critical of doctors than their trained
colleagues. Whether the learners' opinions will change as they
become accustomed to the behaviour of doctors is a moot point. The
general social trend for women to be more assertive and less
submissive is likely to affect nursing to some extent. Briggs suggested
that 'new generations of nurses and midwives share some of the
attitudes of their own generation more than they share the attitudes
of an older generation of nurses and midwives'.[20] However, the
hierarchical systems which seem to flourish in the field of health care
are likely to be very resistant to wider, often hesitant, social
movements. For many nurses consultants are now less often seen as
'gods', they are still seen as being somehow 'up there'.

An examination of the behaviour which some doctors exhibit

towards nurses raises the question as to why nurses tolerate it. Some nurses appear to think doctors have the right to behave in such a fashion. As mentioned earlier, nurses are trained to be submissive. Learners quickly discover that those who speak out are penalized. Most importantly, nurses are taught not to challenge doctors. They are 'schooled into subordination'.[21] There is an inherited image of the nurse as handmaiden to the medical profession.[22] While doctors decide what to do, nurses merely carry out their instructions. (A parallel with an industrial division of labour is made by Dingwall.)[23] Although there are a few nurses at the top who are outspoken and vocal, the majority of nurses are silent. By their silence they allow doctors to be dominant. 'A silent partner, by virtue of her silence, begs to be controlled. And the profession of medicine is happy to honor the request.'[24,25] Of course, other factors are influential. Nurses tend to come from lower socio-economic groups than doctors. It has further been argued that nurses, as women, are a caste within a class.[26] Thus, the power relationships within nursing echo those of the wider society.[27] Doctors dominate because they are men and because they come from a higher socio-economic class.

The sense of superiority that doctors frequently hold is one that is given support from the general public as well as nurses. In comparison with doctors, nurses have fewer qualifications, receive less training and have fewer career prospects. Because nurses often have breaks in their careers, they are felt to have less commitment to their job than doctors. Nurses have less to offer patients (see below) and, of course, nurses are paid less than doctors. Associated with the level of pay is the reduced status and prestige which nurses enjoy when compared with their medical colleagues. Although many nurses enjoy public sympathy and appreciation, they are less respected than members of the medical profession.

Greater respect is bestowed on doctors because they can 'cure' people. Doctors can postpone death, therefore they command both authority and respect.[28] Stereotypes in the mass media appear to enhance the status of doctors at the expense of nurses. Nurses are presented in the media as being less helpful and less empathetic to the needs of patients than doctors.[29] Yet when the reality of nurses' work is considered, the stereotype is revealed for what it is: a put-down of nurses and of women. Male nurses also receive a put-down through being associated with women and women's work. Thus, male nurses are popularly assumed to be homosexual.[30]

A consideration of the range of nurses' work and responsibilities illustrates that they are more than handmaidens of the medical profession. Health visitors, midwives, nurse specialists in intensive care and renal units, in paediatrics, in mental handicap and care of the mentally disturbed are not handmaidens of anybody. They have their own skills, separate and distinct from those of doctors. A part of the problem is the use of the term 'nurse' to cover so many different occupations. However, the fact that the skills of these nurses and midwives are valued less than those of doctors is mainly a reflection of the domination of health care by the primarily male, medical establishment. And where, as in midwifery, the skills of delivery are widely valued by the population at large, we find that there has been a gradual but steady encroachment of the territory of midwives by the medical profession.[31] (Nurses are fighting back. For example, the Cumberlege Report argued for a much enlarged role for nurses in primary health care.)[32] Cumberlege also commissioned a survey which suggested that two-thirds of patients would be prepared to see a nurse instead of a doctor. In some areas of health care the role of doctors is not great, e.g. in relation to the incurable and the dying. Similarly, for the mentally handicapped, the elderly and the disabled, for whom the notion of cure is completely inappropriate, doctors have only a minimal role.

It should not occasion surprise, therefore, that the areas within health care which enjoy greatest prestige are those where the interventions of the medical profession are greatest.[33] At the same time, 'the worst funded areas are, of course, those furthest from the curative process'.[34] Within a Health Service which is dominated by the acute sector, it is apparent that the medical profession occupies centre stage. Doctors tend to disparage the psycho-social aspects of health care which nurses would wish to emphasize.[35] Indeed those courses in medical training such as psychology, sociology[36] which are not mandatory tend to be shunned by medical students. Doctors are taught to prescribe, move on and not to waste their talents on time-consuming bedside care.[37] From the way in which resources are allocated within the Health Service, it is apparent that the 'cure' ethos of doctors completely overshadows the 'care' ethos of nurses. The NHS is geared towards illness rather than health and towards acute health care rather than the needs of the long-term sick. Yet, nursing itself is also geared towards the acute, hospital sector.[38] Recent calls have been made to re-orient nursing towards a preventive role in health care within the community and away from its hospital bias.[39]

As the first-year learners attest, getting used to the position of nurses *vis-à-vis* doctors is not always easy. But these learners enter a ready-made system, developed over decades, in which the dominance of the medical profession has become virtually unassailable. This aspect of 'the System' within which nurses work is of critical importance to everything that nurses do. The way nurses are taught to relate to patients; the tasks which they can and cannot do; their position within the health care team, etc. are all influenced by the dominance of the medical profession. The prestige accorded to doctors in the acute, high intervention sector of health care militates against prestige being accorded to those who work in low-tech, low-intervention sectors. The rankings of prestige amongst the medical profession are reflected in the preferences of nurses. Shortages of nurses, for example, occur particularly in areas such as mental illness, medicine for the elderly, and mental handicap. The areas in which the contribution of nurses is greatest do not enjoy much status amongst nurses. Thus, in the questionnaires, working on surgical wards emerged as the most popular choice of specialty while working in the field of mental illness the least popular. In taking on board received opinion about the importance of cure as distinct from that of care, nurses ensure the continuation of the present relationship with, and dominance of, the medical profession.

As will be seen in later chapters, nurses' self-concept, their relations with other nurses, their attitudes towards trade unions and striking are all influenced by the dominance of the medical profession and its priorities regarding health care.

Nursing itself is changing. But, according to most of the nurses I spoke to, nursing is not changing for the better. (I asked only nurses who had been in post for some time this question.)

In the first place, nurse training has become 'too academic' and increasingly, the wrong type of person is coming into nursing.

> One of the biggest problems is insisting on so many O levels. I don't think its always the best type of girl that has all the O levels and A levels. (Sister)

The opinion that nurses should not be too academic is shared by others:

> I once worked with an anaesthetist for 8 years and he used to say he would sooner have a girl who was really interested in nursing and caring to hold his hand if he was poorly and nurse him, than someone who was all very, very clever and had all the degrees in the world. (Sister)

Being suspicious of the clever nurse, while only admiring of the clever doctor,[40] helps reinforce the view of nurses as being inferior to doctors.[41] Nevertheless, numerous comments about the need for practical rather than academic skills were made.

Secondly, there is said to be less discipline within nursing: nurses speak back and question why they have to do something.

. . . when I started nursing I wouldn't dare speak to a staff nurse.
I certainly wouldn't go through a door in front of a sister . . . I've
discussed it with some of my colleagues and said 'is it me or . . .?'
and they all say that nowadays you can ask learners to do things
and some of them don't like being told. I think the youngsters get
a lot more freedom than they did do. (Staff Nurse)

. . . there's less discipline. From when they start school on day
one they are taught to question things whereas perhaps we
weren't. Perhaps we were a little bit more blind and a little bit
more dumb . . . and if somebody gave you a request or an order
you did it, and you might have a moan about it afterwards, but
you didn't actually question it at the time. (Staff Nurse)

It is not the caricature music-hall battleaxes in the senior ranks of
nursing who make such comments. The emphases on discipline come
from relatively young nurses in their late 20s. These nurses are more
likely to have a teaching role than their more senior colleagues and
have greater contact with the new recruits. As a result they are in a
position to perceive changes in nurse recruits. It may be that their
perception of new recruits ensures they give particular, and influential, emphasis to learners on the need for discipline and respect. They
certainly feel that the young people entering nursing today are more
assertive and less submissive than their older colleagues.

Things have changed so much in the last ten years. In the days
when I was training there was so much respect for your staff
nurses, your sisters: the students and pupils are so confident
now. I don't know if it is a good thing or not. I used to tremble if a
doctor talked to me. If a nursing officer came in I would stand up
until she had gone. (Enrolled nurse)

Thirdly, nursing has become more technical and nursing *care* is
seen by some nurses as losing importance with the result that patient
care suffers.

. . . they are wanting them to go to university and have degrees
and whatever before coming into nursing. And I don't go along
with that. They are too keen on bookwork and not as keen on the
patients. You know they are so highly educated and so well up on
the bookwork, the long words and everything, like the patients
come second, they delegate the work too much rather than
working with the patient, particularly in this type of [psychiatric]
nursing. (Sister)

The reasons given for the changes in nursing are diverse: low-
staffing levels, the many reorganizations within the NHS in recent

years and the introduction of the nursing process.[42] (The nursing process involves individual nurses being assigned to individual patients. Instead of performing the same task for many patients, one nurse will perform most of the tasks for one patient. Nursing becomes patient-centred rather than task-centred.)

> You are spending that much time now having to do paper work that you haven't got time to be with your patients. It's this nursing process system. I personally don't think you need to know everything about a person's past life to help him live in the future. (Staff Nurse)

Many nurses feel entry requirements are now too high resulting in the wrong sort of person coming into nursing. A lack of alternative employment is implicitly, but never explicitly, given as another reason for the presence of 'less committed' recruits. Trained staff often see nursing as being the second choice of occupation of many learners.

> I think they rely too much on people's qualifications rather than their actual ability and caring attitude. I mean they took girls on who didn't have an O level to their name when they started as a student nurse and they were fantastic nurses. They might have struggled a bit with their exams but they knew how to make a patient comfortable. (Sister)

> I think a lot of people are coming into nursing as a second alternative. You know if they can't get to do what they wanted, say they didn't get their A levels to get to university, then they may consider nursing, whereas they wouldn't have considered it as a first option. (Sister)

However not all nurses think nursing is changing for the worse. Some nurses are enthusiastic about improvements in the job and the training. For example, changes have been made in the training syllabus of students of psychiatry and pupils with greater emphasis on working in the community. Similarly, some nurses feel that the role of nurses (or at least staff nurses) has been increased.

> I think the role of the nurse has extended a lot more. I think nurses are having to know a lot more about the actions of various treatments and things rather than just administration. And I think it will change a lot in the future, definitely. (Staff Nurse)

The introduction of the nursing process is seen positively by some nurses, with qualifications:

. . . we hear a lot about the nursing process and everything. We've gone from being task orientated to having a few patients to look after. Now I have to say I like that, if you have got the staff. I feel nurses get to know the patients more . . . I don't know how many people would agree with me but I like the way we are patient orientated now. But in theory its wonderful, in practice it doesn't work always – if you haven't got the staff. (Sister)

Some nurses welcome the greater independence of the new recruits who are aware of their rights and who object to being used as 'fodder' on the wards. Changes in recruitment are also welcomed.

. . . we are getting more mature students. They are a great asset because they have got experience of life. They can relate perhaps more to the patients than an 18-year-old can, so I think they are of great benefit. They have the disadvantage that they worry about their children and they've got home worries, but then I think as a caring profession we should also be caring about our students as well. Caring for ourselves. (Sister)

A few (registered) nurses, felt that the gap between doctors and nurses was narrowing with the omniscience of doctors being questioned.

. . . it's nice that you have a better rapport with the doctors – its a more informal feeling about the atmosphere. I mean most of the doctors who come onto the children's ward, you are on first name terms with them. I remember when I first started and the Sister introduced me to the doctors and it was first names, I just sort of looked flabbergasted, I couldn't believe it! (Staff)

I think nurses have got a lot more to say for themselves and they play a bigger part in the nurse management of patients which I think is a good thing because you are the one who is dealing at first hand with the patients complaints. I don't think we should just sit back and accept what the doctors say as being gospel. (Staff Nurse)

It would be too soon to say that nursing is changing fundamentally. However, changes are being effected. They result from deliberate attempts to change nursing from within. Changes have been made in the emphases and methods of nurse training. Changes have occurred in the demands made of nurses and in the responsibilities they carry (quite apart from the legal responsibilities of nurses). And there have been changes in the managerial roles of nurses. Wider social changes relating to the position of women have also been taking place. However, working as they do within a conservative and hierarchical organization, nurses are seldom at the forefront of any feminist movements. Nevertheless, nurses are not immune to changes in the wider society and, like other women, are starting to question the taken-for-granted systems. Any movement will be slow but it is unlikely that it can be reversed even by a retrenchment to 'traditional' values. Demographic trends and the resulting shortage of potential school-leavers who can be recruited to nursing will give clout to the women who are nurses. The impending shortage of nurses means they will be in relatively powerful positions to obtain improvements in their working lives. Some idea of the type of improvements that nurses would presently like to see made will be given in later chapters.

For the moment however, changes which *negatively* affect nurses, especially those with domestic commitments, are still taking place. Nurses are being asked to rotate onto night duty at periodic intervals. No longer will nurses be able to work 'fixed nights'. At the moment some nurses on night duty elect to work on the same 2 or 3 nights each week. There also appears to have been a reduction in the amount of part-time nursing work which is available. There is, obviously, no immediate shortage of nurses in this district health authority.

As this chapter and the previous one have shown there is 'a system' waiting to receive the nurse recruit. It is a system which is set in its ways. It seems to be a system which is unchallengeable by individuals. Yet, as will be seen in Chapter 11, it is a system which is currently facing far-reaching changes. 'The system' will change.

Notes

1 For an account of the way in which men came into nursing see Dingwall, R. (1979) 'The place of men in nursing' *in* Colledge, M. and Jones, D. (eds) *A Reader in Nursing*, Edinburgh, Churchill Livingstone.
2 See Brown, R.G.S. and Stones, R.W.H. (1973) *The Male Nurse* London, Bell, pp. 21–3; Harrison and Gretton (eds) (1984) p. 111.
3 Hardy, L.K. (1984) 'The emergence of nursing leaders – a case of in-spite of, not because-of', *International Nursing Review*, 31:1, p.13.
4 See Waite, R. and Hutt, R. (1987), p. 70. This research was confined to members of the Royal College of Nursing.
5 See Salvage (1985), p. 10.
6 Simpson and Simpson *in* Etzioni (ed) (1969), p. 229.
7 Gaze, H. (1987) 'Man Appeal', *Nursing Times*, 20 May, 83, 30, p. 25; Hardy, L. (1987) 'The Male Model', *Nursing Times*, 27 May, 83:21, pp. 36–8.
8 It has also been argued that the changes introduced as a result of the recommendations of the Salmon Committee published in 1966 for more professional management acted so as to favour men (see Carpenter 'Managerialism and the division of labour in nursing' (1978) *in* Dingwall and McIntosh, pp. 98–9).

9 See Harrison and Gretton (1984), p. 111.

10 For some idea of the numbers of nurses working outside the NHS in various areas and institutions, see Department of Health and Social Security (1982) *Nurse Manpower: Maintaining the Balance*, London, DHSS, p. 81.

11 See Wright, S. (1985) 'New nurses: new boundaries', *Nursing Practice* 1:1, p. 33.

12 ibid. p. 33.

13 Salvage (1985) op cit., p. 171.

14 Women continue to be very much in the minority within the ranks of qualified doctors – see Merrison (1979), p. 170, but the number of women medical undergraduates and GP trainees has increased considerably since the mid-70s – see the White Paper (1987) *Promoting Better Health*, London, HMSO, Cm. 249, p. 20.

15 See Duncan and McLachlan, G. (1984), p. 19.

16 However, situations do arise where doctors take advice from nurses, albeit in a roundabout fashion. See, for example, Keddy, B., Jones, M., Jacobs, P., Burton, H. and Rogers, M. (1986) 'The doctor-nurse relationship: an historical perspective' *Journal of Advanced Nursing*. 11:6, pp. 745–53; and Hughes, D. (1988) 'When nurse knows best: some aspects of nurse/doctor interaction in a casualty department'. *Sociology of Health and Illness*, March, 10:1, pp. 1–22.

17 The British Medical Association and the RCN have been described as having a 'growing battle' regarding preventive health care as a result of the recommendations of the Cumberlege Report – P. Hilldrew (1986) 'Nurses fighting GPs for power', *The Guardian*, 21 July, p. 4.

18 See Wright (1985), p. 33.

19 Mitchell, R.G. *in* Duncan and McLachlan (eds) (1984), p. 54.

20 DHSS (1972), p. 28.

21 Gaze (1987), p. 27.

22 See DHSS (1972), p. 23.

23 Carpenter *in* Dingwall and McIntosh (eds) (1978) Chapter 6.

24 Lovell, M.C. (1981) 'Silent but perfect 'partners': medicine's use and abuse of women', *Advances in Nursing Science*, 3:1, p. 27.

25 For a discussion of the position of nurses vis-a-vis the medical profession, see Darbyshire, P. (1987) 'The burden of history' *Nursing Times*, 28 January, 83:4, pp. 32–4, Ehrenreich and English (1973), Gaze (1987), Lovell (1981).

26 Lovell (1981), p. 27.

27 Darbyshire (1987), p. 32.

28 See Wright (1985); Darbyshire (1987); Etzioni (ed) (1969).

29 Kalisch, P.A. and Kalisch, B.J. (1986) 'A comparative analysis of nurse and physician characters in the entertainment media'. *Journal of Advanced Nursing*, 11:2, p. 189 – the authors describe the presentation of nurses and doctors in the media. Although the research relates to the USA, many programmes from the USA are, and have been, seen in this country.

30 For a pithy rejoinder to such charges, see Lawrence, J.C. (1978) 'Male nurses: a different view', *Imprint*, 25:1, pp. 28–30.

31 The numbers of home confinements are continuing to decrease as are the

numbers of midwives working in the community (see Merrison (1979), p. 78). In the UK, 80 per cent of births take place in hospital compared with 2 per cent in Holland (Tuckett *in* Tuckett (ed.) (1976), p. 377). The World Health Organization showed a very high level of technological intervention in UK compared with most other European countries (World Health Organization (1986) *Having a Baby in Europe*, Geneva, WHO). Concern about the erosion of the role of the midwife is being expressed by many practising midwives (see Brooks, F., Long, A. and Rathwell, T. (1987) *Midwives' Perceptions on the State of Midwifery*, University of Leeds, Nuffield Centre for Health Services Studies, p. 8).

32 Cumberlege, J. (1986) *Neighbourhood Nursing – a Focus for Care*, London, HMSO.
33 The merit awards distributed to consultants by consultants clearly reflect the prestige ratings given to the 'glamorous' areas of health care – Brindle, D. (1988b) 'Pay and privilege on trial', *The Guardian* 18 May p. 4.
34 Davidson (1987) p. 8.
35 Kalisch, B.J. and Kalisch, P. (1977) 'An analysis of the sources of physician–nurse conflict' *Journal of Nursing Administration*, 7:1, p. 54.
36 Darbyshire (1987), p. 33.
37 Ehrenreich and English (1973), p. 39.
38 See RCN (1986), p. 7.
39 Promoting Better Health (1987) London, HMSO, Cm 249.
40 See Chapman, C.M. (1977) 'Image of the nurse' *International Nursing Review*, 24, p. 166.
41 It is interesting that doctors writing in the *Nursing Times* can object to nurses 'collecting letters behind their name' when that is precisely what helps advance a doctor's career – Devlin, B. (1987) 'An unreal brave new world?', *Nursing Times*, 6 May, 83:18, pp. 29–30.
42 For a description of the nursing process see De La Cuesta, C. (1983) 'The nursing process: from development to implementation' *Journal of Advanced Nursing*, 8, p. 365–71.

5

Constraints on the Job

Nursing work is demanding, stressful, responsible work. This is currently being intensified through the increasing use of 'tight' staffing levels. The skills of nurses are being under-used in an attempt by management to meet the growing demands for cost-effectiveness. The short-term gains are at the expense of the long-term. Levels of stress are felt to be rising by nurses at the same time as morale is falling. Nurses have protected themselves with the idea of their own vocation but the rising amount of absence tells its own story. Nurses are being pushed too far. It seems they are still seen as primarily a female and therefore easily replaceable workforce – a mistake in the light of demographic forecasts.

Nursing is an occupation which is overwhelmingly female in composition. In our society caring is primarily done by women. In the popular stereotypes nursing is women's work. But closer examination reveals that nursing is not what is normally associated with the 'weaker sex'. 'Their work involves carrying out tasks which, by ordinary standards, are distasteful, disgusting and frightening.'[1] Nursing is hard work: physically and mentally tiring and carries the risk of injury. It is often a responsible job which also makes many emotional demands on nurses.

On the other hand, nursing offers intrinsic satisfactions. However, there are many constraints within nursing which affect the experience of work. Some constraints are inherent in the very nature of the job while others are externally imposed. There is a discrepancy between what nurses want to do and what they can do.

Nursing *is* different from other jobs. At least nurses think it is different from other jobs they have had. Nursing is hard work. Indeed,

the life expectancy of a 45-year-old nurse is only 1 year greater than
that of a miner.[2] Nursing is an extremely demanding job:

> You have to give a lot more emotionally. You just can't go and do
> it and that's it – it's not like an office job. You are responsible for
> lives really, which is a lot to ask. (Staff Nurse)
>
> . . . it's not just mentally stressful, the nurses go home mentally
> and physically shattered. Even sometimes the doctors, they were
> in here this morning having a pleasant chat and drinking coffee
> because they had a quiet spell but we never have a quiet spell, to
> sit down, you know. I can't remember the last time I sat down
> and actually talked to a patient, when I wasn't doing something
> for them. (Staff Nurse)

There is a particular stress in the amount of responsibility which
many nurses carry:

> You are the first line of defence, you are. You have to be able to
> resuscitate a baby. If things go wrong, you're thinking 'what else
> can I try before the doctor comes, is there anything else I can
> try?' . . . On night duty you are the only sister and there is
> nobody else on the unit that you can turn to because nobody else
> knows what to do, only you. (Sister)

Nursing is not a job that can be 'walked away from'. Nurses go home
and worry. They worry about things they might have forgotten to do,
the patient they didn't have time to talk to, special instructions on one
thing or another.

> I think it affects your whole life, totally. Your social life – how you
> are with other people. (Student)
>
> . . . you can't walk away at 5 o'clock; there is still a bit of it that
> comes through no matter how much you try and say no . . . I
> think you bring it home with you . . . You get so involved with
> your patient care that you are taking them home and you are
> trying to live their entire life. (Sister)
>
> If I've worked a late duty, I don't particularly sleep that night
> because there are still things racing around. I can't switch off.
> (Sister)

The responsibilities of nursing particularly affected sisters and
charge nurses: not just the newly appointed but older and experienced
nurses as well. While youth and inexperience may make coping with
responsibility particularly stressful,[3] the responsibilities of patients'
lives weigh heavily on many nurses. Nurses are given a great deal of

responsibility when they are very young. There are not many jobs in which 20- or 21-year-olds are left in sole charge (even if help is only a couple of minutes away) of a ward full of patients. Things do go wrong, sudden crises occur and the response of the nurse in charge is often critical. A panicking nurse is no use to anyone. And there is always the fear if you don't do the right thing then a patient's life may well be at risk, even lost.

> A lot of responsibility is given to a lot of very young people. You can be a staff nurse in charge of a ward at 21 being in charge of 24 or 28 people. And having to make life and death decisions – at 21 that's hard. (Sister)

Dealing with people while they are under stress and in sensitive situations calls for both patience and tolerance. This aspect was mentioned by a few nurses. As a corollary to this, some nurses mentioned that it is not a job that you can be half-hearted about:

> To be a nurse you've really got to like it. You can't go into nursing if you think 'I can do it, it will look good . . .'. (Enrolled Nurse)

And at the same time one or two nurses mentioned that nursing is something that they had become addicted to. Subsumed under these comments is a belief in the idea of a vocation. It was an idea which started to be voiced by the learners as they faced the early months of nurse training. The idea of vocation helps counteract the response of nurses to unsavoury tasks. If there is something you dislike doing whether it is emptying colostomy bags or sitting with an unconscious patient, the task becomes less onerous if you can comfort yourself with the knowledge that others could not do it. The only reason that you can do such a task is because you have a vocation. Menzies[4] has argued that the notion of vocation is invoked when ordinary job satisfaction cannot be expected. Many of the duties of nurses are potentially distasteful. Indeed, many patients will tell nurses that they could not do a nurse's job. The 'specialness' of the person who can do the job is not to be denied. To have a vocation is to be a special kind of person.

But, nursing can be seen as a strange job. Most of us choose to spend our lives with the healthy. To have to look after a sick relative or friend is often seen as being burdened. Yet, nurses choose to spend their working lives with ill or disabled people.

> . . . it is a strange job, an unnatural job – dealing with ill people all the time, dealing with disabled people all the time. If you

actually look at yourself and ask 'why did I want to look after
people who are ill?' there isn't a good reason other than caring
and wanting to make them better. (Sister)

Working as a nurse often entails shiftwork, working at weekends
and during the night. Hardly surprisingly, shifts are not universally
liked by nurses. Most nurses prefer some shifts to others. Preferences
often reflect the domestic commitments. Most popular is the 'early'
shift starting around 7 a.m. and finishing in mid-afternoon. Night
shift is least liked but nearly a fifth of questionnaire respondents
preferred it.

There is a wide variety of shift patterns working amongst nurses.
Community nurses often work an ordinary 8-hour day but be 'on call'
during the evening or over the weekend. Nurses in the psychiatric
hospital work 12-hour shifts, but the shift pattern was predictable and
nurses knew their rota well in advance. In general hospital nursing,
in contrast, a nurse may be asked at extremely short notice to work
'split shifts' or to change shift the next day. Split shifts, that is working
half an 'early' shift and half a 'late' shift, are not much liked. The
inconvenience of shifts is sometimes mentioned as THE factor which
had made a nurse think about leaving:

> I do like the job. Some days it does get you down. Saturdays and
> Sundays when you are at work and everyone else is home.
> You've got to structure yourself around the shift system and your
> pay as well. At the end of the month you look at your pay slip and
> think what you have done, for this! (Student)

Being asked to change shifts at short notice seldom happens now.
However, when nurses report in for work they are sometimes moved
because of a staff shortage to another ward due to sickness or
absence. Rather than bring in 'bank' nurses, nurse managers try to
'make do' with the nurses they already have in the hospital. (Bank
nurses are nurses who are on the books of the hospital, rather in the
same way as the private nursing agencies operate. The only difference
being that bank nurses work for the NHS.) Nurses do not relish being
moved onto another ward.

> I don't particularly like it, reason being that you just feel as
> though you're a pair of hands – you're just told to go and work on
> another unit. You don't know who's who or what's the matter
> with them. If a doctor comes onto the ward and says can I see Mrs
> such-and-such and you've got to get out a piece of paper or come
> into the office to find out . . . you are just a bit clueless and you
> feel incompetent really. (Staff Nurse)

Nurses may not like being moved but it is fast becoming just another part of the job. Given the pressures on nurse managers not to spend more money, they have little alternative but to try to cope with the nurses they've got. However, there are undoubted strains on the nursing workforce in covering for their absent colleagues.

Over half the nurses who completed a questionnaire felt absence was a problem. A third said absence was 'sometimes' a problem. Through absenteeism, extra pressure is put on the staff who do turn up for work. When staffing levels are already felt to be low, absence puts greater pressure on the others. It causes low morale and resentment. Nurse managers are left having to shuffle nurses from one place to another. They are well aware of nurses' dislike of being moved around, yet their hands are tied. Absence is a problem for nurse managers and for nurses.[5] Absence is a self-perpetuating problem. The more nurses who do not report in for work, the greater the pressure on the nurses who do. The more intense the pressure on nurses, the greater the strain they feel. As the strains of nursing mount, nurses feel less and less like turning up for work. Being absent becomes 'normal' and an accepted response to the pressures of nursing.[6]

It is almost irrelevant whether nurses are really ill or whether they just want a day off from the strains of nursing. Whether its physical illness or mental and emotional strain the result is the same – a nurse short for duty that day.

In a way you can't blame them because if you are persistently working with the minimum amount of staff then you're bound to get over-tired and you get your days off and you just collapse and you don't feel refreshed when you get back to work and you do feel rundown. (Sister)

. . . I think its increasing and I'm sure its some of the workload they have to cope with; and, as the staffing levels get lower you have more to do. Probably once upon a time they might have shrugged it off and gone to work . . . (Sister)

You understand really when others go off sick because you know you're trying to do your best and then you're making yourself ill – you're really working hard. You know, you're substituting for somebody else who has gone off sick so you do their work and then the week after you're off sick because you can't cope. (Enrolled Nurse)

A persistent thread running through the comments on absence is that of the already 'tight' staffing levels. Nurses feel that their numbers have been cut to the minimum possible. Absence rates are seen to be high by nurses, e.g. 'its never been as bad'. However from statistics collected from one of the hospitals concerned it is not clear that absence is an increasing problem. Indeed, the absence rates seem to be just below the national average for nursing staff in the health service. Absence is perceived as a greater problem by nurses than it is because of the already tight staffing levels. But absence is a quiet way of indicating discontent. By arguing the growing importance of absence nurses demonstrate their own disenchantment with nursing in the NHS. Unwilling to take visible and collective action, absence is obviously one of the few courses open if you need to keep your job yet wish to register complaint.

According to many nurses the heart of the problem is understaffing. Not all specialties are understaffed. Some specialist units have few, if any, problems regarding staffing levels. Difficulties seem to be encountered on units which involve particularly heavy work. For example, medical or geriatric wards are 'heavy' in that there is a lot of lifting of patients to be done. Nursing stroke patients involves 'the back round': turning patients every two hours in order to avoid pressure sores. It is an onerous job much complained about by learners to whom the task often seems to fall. And it is from such hard and heavy work that nurses are more likely to go off 'sick'. But in other specialties the staffing levels are reasonable:

> I think we are probably one of the better staffed wards because they tend to need more staff for the burns patients. We are quite well staffed. I mean there's times when you think you should have more staff but I think compared to the medical wards we are not too badly off. (Staff Nurse)

On paper, the staffing levels are probably adequate. In reality with one nurse off sick here and one on maternity leave there, staffing becomes less than adequate. Six out of the seven nursing officers I spoke to made such a point.

> If everybody is in and everybody is working . . . But there isn't a week when it's like that – very rarely anyway. Every member of staff gets seven weeks with the bank holidays, and maternity leave, sickness – there's always somebody off.

A factor complicating staffing levels in one hospital was that the wards were designed on a system of bays rather than the traditional Nightingale ward. Keeping an eye on the patients is much harder in the bay system. On a Nightingale ward a nurse can glance down the ward to check that everyone is all right. With bays, nurses have to walk round and check each bay. If only a few nurses are on duty, it is difficult to find time to stop what you are doing and go round. If patients are not continuously checked, accidents can and do happen.

> I don't like the bays because you just cannot see your patients. Nightingale wards are much better – you can see if someone is going to fall out of bed. The side bays are miles away from the office. Some call them 'Siberia' – you cannot keep an eye on them properly. Some patients do fall out of bed. It's bad really. These are the cases that come out in the papers. (Staff Nurse)

It is not clear whether the Regional Health Authority takes account of the ward design in the staffing levels it allows. The DHSS can warn that guidelines on staffing norms 'should be used with caution and examined in the light of local circumstances'.[7] However, when extreme financial pressures are being put on district health authorities to curtail costs, it is not easy to use such guidelines with caution. Pleas regarding special local circumstances are likely to be heard from all directions and hardly excite much sympathy.

In some specialties staffing levels present particular difficulties because demand cannot be predicted. There is no way of knowing whether there will be a major traffic accident or how many heart attack victims there will be on any one morning. With the best possible planning there will be discrepancies, either too many or too few nurses.

> . . . the last two nights we've had somebody with a head injury who has needed somebody to sit by him all the time, and it's just impossible. There's no spare people, that's the problem. You can manage so long as everything is fine, but the moment you get a real emergency or anything . . . (Student)

Overall it appears that staffing levels are tight. There is little 'slack' to be taken up when nurses go absent or sick. And when nurses take maternity leave replacements are seldom made.

> . . . when we have anyone on maternity leave they are not replaced. They just say 'well, they are being paid while they are on maternity leave, there is no more money to pay somebody else'. So we all have to get round that bit more. And, when I was off for three months, nobody else came in – it was just coped with by the people who were there, which isn't awfully fair. (District Nurse)

Even *before* a nurse goes on maternity leave there are problems:

> . . . not very long ago we had two SENs pregnant and a learner

pregnant as well, so we were carrying them all – because they
can't lift or anything on the ward, and it's very heavy. (Staff
Nurse)

Nurses have to be particularly careful when they are pregnant.
Lifting patients is heavy work and quite a number of nurses are
injured at work. Over a third of the questionnaire nurses had injured
themselves at work. Back injuries accounted for half the injuries the
nurses sustained while a fifth of nurses had been assaulted by
patients.[8] Another quarter of nurses had sustained an injury to a limb,
e.g. twisted ankle, broken arm.[9] Not every injury causes a nurse to go
home. Indeed, in some units, nurses seemed to soldier on regardless,
with perhaps some degree of pride:

> . . . they have a little thing there that it's disprin and crutches,
> you are not allowed to be off sick. They've made a joke of it there.
> It's a different attitude from a different nursing officer. I mean
> there were days I went in and I was being sick four or five times,
> but I wouldn't dream not to go just because I was being sick
> because I was pregnant. (Staff Nurse)

No attempt was made to determine whether or not injury levels had
changed in the last few years. However, a few nurses made the link
between the numbers of injury and staffing levels. When you are only
too aware of how busy you are and how busy your colleagues are, you
don't interrupt them to ask them to come and help you lift a heavy
patient. You try to do it on your own, against the strictures of training
and repeated warnings not to.

> When you are lifting you should have two people. I had to lift a
> patient and I called for help and when the SEN came she was not
> happy with me. She said she would have lifted the patient on her
> own. I said I wouldn't advise her to do it on her own. (Student)

From the number of back injuries it is obvious that many nurses do
lift patients on their own. They do it until they hurt themselves. Back
injury seems to happen most frequently when trying to move a
patient up the bed, getting them to sit up. There appears to be
resistance amongst some nurses to using the lifting aids which are
available. Such aids may be seen as 'more bother than they are
worth'. It has also been argued that nurses' uniforms and the design
of hospital beds are inappropriate for the lifting that nurses do and
exacerbating the number of back injuries.[10]

However, pressure of work, of trying to get through all the jobs that
have to be done seems to be the major contributing factor. Lifting a
patient alone is a costly practice: to the nurse who is injured and to

the health authority. It is just another repercussion from the tight staffing levels in the NHS.

Two-thirds of the questionnaire 'stayers' felt their workload had increased in the previous 12 months. Over a third said their workload was 'more' and just under a third said that their workload was 'much more'. The nurses I spoke to corroborated these findings. Of course, workload is subject to fluctuations. Some wards and units are busier than others. Some days and weeks are busier than others.

> It varies on here, sometimes you are only 10–15 per cent full; sometimes you're absolutely boiling over. I would say over the last year, the workload here has increased. We're getting a lot more chronic people, people with long-standing behavioural problems and things like that. (Staff Nurse)

A few nurses positively enjoyed the increased workload, and some nurses themselves sought a heavier workload:

> My workload is heavy through choice, and I take a lot more on than I actually need to, but if I chose not to do that, I don't think there would be any complaints about it. (Sister)

Other nurses complained of not being busy enough:

> I have lost a lot of patients with the 'zoning' and I've never gained from anywhere else. So I'm not as busy as I was . . . Its very frustrating, especially when you know other clinics are busy. It takes away a bit of the satisfaction of the job. (District Nurse)

Some nurses had changed jobs in the previous 12 months, going to work in a different unit or area, and their workload had changed:

> It was heavier when I worked on the wards . . . but down here we try and get it on a one-to-one basis. They need a lot of doing so it's more intense but not as heavy. You are not as tired at the end of the day: psychologically rather than physically tiring. (Staff Nurse).

However, for the majority of nurses the workload had increased and it was not a welcome increase. This appears to be only a part of a continuing intensification of the work of nurses. Briggs, for example, in 1972 commented that due to earlier discharges 'within hospitals the pace, pressure and intensity of work have stepped up because a greater proportion of the patients are in need of active treatment. It has also meant that the quantity and nature of the burden carried by the community nursing services has altered markedly.'[11]

The greater workload reported by the nurses I talked to was put down to a variety of reasons: staffing levels, more paperwork, a decrease in the number of learners, and cutting back on the number of ancillary staff.

> I started here 12 months ago in January and there were a lot of staff. Well, there weren't more staff, there were a lot more learners, which makes a big difference obviously. (Staff Nurse)

> Yes, staff are leaving and not being replaced. We are doing more jobs that we shouldn't be doing . . . They've cut back on things like the domestics. When we don't have one we have to do it ourselves. Well it takes you away from your nursing care, your patients – it's all the extra things that you are having to do. (Staff Nurse)

Nurses appear to regularly carry out tasks which should properly be carried out by others: domestics, social workers, doctors, etc. (see Appendix 9).[12]

Having to do the work of other grades of staff is not simply a case of having more work. It means that nurses do not spend their time nursing. It can also mean that less time is spent with the patients. If nurses are doing the work of more senior personnel then there is likely to be added responsibility and added stress in carrying out duties for which they may not feel themselves adequately prepared. And if nurses are carrying out the duties of less senior personnel then they are not using their skills. It also involves a waste of resources if expensively trained nurses are doing the work of catering and domestic staff.[13] The training of learners can also be negatively affected. Thus learners, in their second and third years, complained about having to do a good deal of non-nursing work:

> On the geriatric ward that I was on, we just seemed to spend the whole time cleaning the ward and we complained about that. I realize that you have to do non-nursing duties, but it's when it takes over from your learning that I don't agree with it. We didn't get any teaching sessions on that ward – nothing at all. (Student)

The shortage of ancillary staff was often blamed directly on 'government cuts' in NHS funding. At the same time the advancing privatization of laundry and cleaning services was a cause for concern.

> When we moved to this hospital they cut the hours of the domestics. They are going to bring in private people now. But are they going to expect the nurses in the future to do some of the cleaning? The qualified nurses I mean – it's not fair to expect them to clean. We'll have to wait and see. (Sister)

Given the above findings that nurses often do the work of others, it is not surprising that many nurses feel their skills and talents are being under-used.[14] It seems that nurses are increasingly being used as 'a pair of hands'. Using a skilled workforce to do the jobs of cleaners or messengers is quite clearly a false economy. There may be short-term economic gains but there are likely to staffing problems in the longer-term if the skilled workforce leave as a result. Similarly, the fact that nurses have to carry out so many and such a range of tasks which are not central to nursing care, may produce real difficulties in maintaining standards of patient care. In simple terms understaffing leads to the deskilling of nursing. Thus most nurses are increasingly engaged in carrying out menial tasks. For a select few, highly qualified or specialized, nursing will continue to be challenging and rewarding. For the rest, however, understaffing means unrewarding and un-challenging work. If the calibre of recruits to nursing is lowered in response to the present experiences of nursing work, a division between the ranks and officers within nursing may be created. Thus, there may come to be a middle-class career nurse and a working-class menial assistant. Such a division may, of course, already be in sight with the elimination of the enrolled nurse grade and the creation of the 'helper' (see Chapter 11).

Nursing is a stressful job. The vast majority of nurses found nursing stressful. There are many components to this experience of stress[15] such as staff shortages, the level of responsibility, dealing with death and the dying, patients' relatives, and coping with unpredictable patients.

Staff shortages and their effects emerged as being the single most important cause of stress. The responsibility for patients' wellbeing can be onerous.

Responsibility to and for patients is accompanied (for those in charge) with responsibility for the staff and learners.

> I don't feel it so much now, but when I qualified at 22, having twenty-seven patients' lives in my hands when I'm being in charge . . . I mean there's a lot of back-up on here, they all say phone me up at home, you can phone the consultants any time you want, but sort of walking out on to the ward and you've got the learners underneath you, so if they do anything wrong it's you, if anything happens on the ward then it's you, and you've got to look after your patients but double-check on all your staff, double check on all your doctors and I think that's part of it, I don't think you can ever relax. (Staff Nurse)

Nursing is emotionally stressful. Dealing with dying patients and

their relatives could never be an easy task. When it is remembered
how young many nurses are, it is salutory to think of the experiences
they have to face in their everyday work. 'Nurses are confronted with
the threat and the reality of suffering and death as few lay people
are.'[16] How many other young people are asked to contend with such
a reality? Even other health-care professionals such as doctors do not
have to face, as nurses do, the stressful situation of 'intimate contact
with suffering patients'.[17]

When the nurses were asked what caused them the most stress in
their jobs, dealing with the harsher facts of life was often mentioned:

> What upsets me is if we have people of my age in and they die,
> when they are near my age . . . What annoys me is that you
> don't seem to have enough time to do everything . . . (Sister in
> her late 20s)

> There have been times when we have had four children, RTAs
> [road traffic accidents] or whatever, and the prognosis is poor for
> three of them – it can be very stressful. You have a lot of intense
> relatives, they are very tense people. It's distressing to others and
> it distresses you to see the other people distressed. And everybody
> seems to get to a fever pitch . . . (Staff Nurse)

> . . . on the labour ward if something has gone wrong, if the
> baby's born flat and getting the baby resuscitated – that's quite
> stressful because you've got to act really quickly to get things
> right . . . Or having to deal with a child that's born with
> congenital abnormalities or still births – that's quite emotional
> really. (Staff Nurse)

> I think its probably an NAI [non-accidental injury to a child] or a
> sick baby. Sometimes you don't get a lot of support from the
> doctor, he won't go out and he tells you to go out. We are not
> trained to diagnose, we are not supposed to do it. You are very
> frightened if you miss something – a baby might not look very ill
> but . . . (Health Visitor)

> I think really when a patient asks you 'Am I dying?' and you
> can't say 'yes' if they are, when they obviously are. I would like to
> put those barriers aside and talk about what is to come ahead if
> they are going to die. I think that should be pushed a bit more –
> how to cope with that. (Staff Nurse)

The most stressful moments for nurses are what might be called
'unfair deaths' and 'unfair illness': children and young adults who are
dying, babies who have been battered and uncared for. They are
patients who somehow ought not to be there.

The nurses' comments illustrate the way in which the already heavy burden of looking after very ill patients is exacerbated by other factors. The additional contraints imposed by 'the system' or other professionals are easier to 'sound off' about than complaining about the demands of dying, and helpless, patients. While the demands of patients are an integral part of the job, the constraints imposed by others may sometimes be 'the last straw' to a nurse facing a stressful situation.

Pressure is also present due to the increasing threat of litigation. Only a minority of nurses mentioned it, but for some the possibility of legal action is worrying. It is yet another reflection of the responsibility which nurses have to carry.

> One of the things at the moment which is growing is the possibility of being sued. It's good in a way because it keeps you on your toes, but it also does put more pressure on you as well. (Staff Nurse)

The experience of stress varies with grade, specialty[18] and location. Although staff shortages were mentioned by all grades of nurses, they were less often mentioned by sisters and psychiatric nurses. For sisters, outside psychiatry, dealing with death was the most stressful aspect. Junior nurses are likely to have greater contact in their day-to-day work with the dying patient. However, sisters have more contact with patients' relatives, breaking the news of recent or impending death and dealing with relatives' distress. In psychiatry on the other hand, there are different stresses.

> The assessment ward is hard. Patients are admitted from home and they are all very restless and if you want to get the best out of them you have to cut the drugs down. That makes them more restless, so you have a physical as well as a mental stress. (Sister)

For nurses at all levels, but in particular for staff nurses, stress was due to the amount of responsibility:

> I think it's the decision-making and the responsibility you carry. Obviously you work as a team and then you have to take decisions as a team. But sometimes you have to take decisions on your own and you need to be confident about what you are doing. (Staff Nurse)

Sisters, on the other hand, mentioned 'the responsibility' on fewer occasions than other grades. The weight of responsibility which they felt was having to deal with, and respond to, emergencies.

   . . . you do have people's lives in your hands – you come across
   so many emergency situations and you've got to be on the ball all
   the time. So your brain is sort of ticking . . . (Sister)

It is interesting that quite a high proportion of enrolled nurses and
learners (about a fifth) also mentioned responsibility as being an
important aspect of their stress. It is not simply whether nurses ARE
responsible which is influential, but whether they FEEL responsible
which matters.

   There are many other aspects of nurses' jobs which may be
experienced as stressful such as the amount of driving required in the
community nurse's job, having to assist in administering ECT against
one's own beliefs in the psychiatric nurse's job, the degree of
involvement required in looking after the mentally handicapped, etc.

   While nursing is stressful for many nurses it is not that aspect they
most often moan about. The stressfulness of nursing seems to be
accepted as part of the job.

   I don't think you would be a good nurse unless you have got a
   certain amount of stress. Because if we ever got used to seeing
   people dying, if you ever got blasé about it or anything like that,
   you couldn't comfort relatives, you just couldn't. (District Nurse)

I asked the nurses what they would most likely be moaning about
when they got home. One or two nurses had no complaints: 'I
couldn't moan about nursing really' (Enrolled Nurse). But for the
majority there were numerous complaints of which understaffing was
the most frequently expressed. Throughout the conversations with
the nurses understaffing was a constantly recurring theme. Understaffing is felt in many different ways in the daily work experience of
nurses. It affects the pace and quality of work. Nurses complain about
declining standards, of not having enough time to talk to patients or
be with patients when they are needed. Both tasks and patients are
rushed.

   I used to get very upset by the fact that I could work from quarter
   to eight to five, do without my dinner hour, work to the full and
   do the best I could and still know that a lot of patients didn't get
   any care, you know the care they should have done or needed.
   (Staff Nurse)

Nurses work overtime and seldom seem to get their 'time back'.
Payment is not given for working past finishing time. Instead time off
in lieu is meant to be taken. That is not as straightforward as it
appears. When you know your colleagues are struggling to get all the

work done, it is not easy to say you're wanting the time off that you are due. And working beyond finishing time can be a frequent occurrence.

> On ward X – that used to be very, very frustrating, because I would never get time back. Many nights when I was in charge it would be twenty to six when I was getting off which wasn't so bad at odd times. But when it happened time and time again, I used to find that really frustrating. (Student)

Working late is just a reflection of the workload which many nurses bear. And moans about workload are frequently voiced.

> I don't really moan – only that I'm tired and I feel as though I've got too much on and I've got a queue of people outside waiting to see me, and yes . . . but what I normally say is 'if I had 48 hours in today, I'd be all right'. Or if somebody would cut the wires on the telephone for me. (Sister)

Given the moans about understaffing and workload it is not surprising that many nurses talk of standards going down.

> One confused lady who can't manage to control her bowels shouldn't have a ratty nurse because she's overworked and she knows that the rest are sat in wet knickers because they can't get to the toilet, its not . . . (Staff Nurse)

Other aspects are moaned about: pay (which will be looked at in greater detail in Chapter 6) and relations with other nurses (which is discussed in Chapter 7). Interestingly, the way in which nurses react to one another is easily the biggest moan amongst the learners but it was less often complained about by the trained nurses.

Sadly, nurses felt that morale within their hospital or specialty was none too high. Morale was lowest in the large, new general hospital. At the time the shock waves of one hospital amalgamating with another were just beginning to die down. Old divisions and distinctions were fondly remembered. Some staff seemed to positively relish, by avidly recounting, the ostensibly 'poor' practices of their newer colleagues. Some 6 months later, there was some evidence that things were settling down. Nevertheless, morale was still not high. A particular and insuperable problem was that of size. The hospital was thought to be too big and hence felt to be too anonymous by most nurses – many of whom had been transferred from much smaller hospitals. The medical facilities of the general hospital were generally held to be excellent and there was some pride in this. However, the design of the wards, mentioned earlier, caused a great deal of discontent. The bay system could have been accommodated more easily if staffing levels were less tight. The nursing management were caught in a dilemma not of their own making. They had to bring in potentially hostile nurses to a new hospital where staffing levels were 'efficient'. Nursing management was stuck with a hospital size and ward design which it probably would not have chosen.

The result has been a nursing workforce which has been slow to settle down in a large hospital with long corridors and wards in which nurses have to keep on the move. In some respects it is surprising that morale is not lower.

Morale in the other hospitals and services was found to be fair. There was disquiet in the mental hospital which was scheduled for closure in the early 1990s. Staff were uncertain about their own and their patients' future. Having said that, the hospital was a self-contained community which appeared to offer a lot of support to its members. For the nurses working in the community and mental-handicap services morale appeared to be improving.

Morale, of course, is a nebulous concept: impossible to quantify[19] and to pin down to specific concerns. Currently, morale is not felt to be high amongst nurses generally.[20] Kogan has suggested that morale relates more to 'general feelings about the NHS than to feelings of satisfaction with their jobs of working context'.[21] Nevertheless, local conditions and constraints must affect nurses' view of morale amongst their colleagues. Low morale is perhaps best equated with an atmosphere of grumbling. Thus, when two nurses meet and exchange pleasantries, they expect to hear grumbles about this or that. It is a self-reinforcing process, a spiral out of which it is extremely difficult to break. But it is a problem which must be faced by nurse managers and not ignored on the grounds that they didn't know what 'morale' actually was (a sentiment expressed on a number of occasions by senior nurses in the health authority). After all, high morale amongst nursing staff has been shown, by Revans, to hasten the recovery of patients.[22] Similarly, low morale is likely to spill over into nurses' attitudes towards patients[23] as can stress.[24]

The list of complaints which has been recited in this chapter should not disguise the fact that many nurses are very happy with their jobs. Everyone moans about their job at some time. Most of us can manage to compile quite a long list of petty irritations at work. Some nurses feel strongly about one aspect, some about another. There is only one topic which rises above all others in importance and it is that of staffing levels. The majority of nurses feel that if staffing levels were improved than many of their grouses and moans would disappear. Nurses would have an easier workload, absence and sickness might be reduced, injuries at work might go down, nurses might be moved around less, if only there were more nurses. There would be less need to do the work of others, the talents and skills of nurses would be properly used, much of the stress of the job would go – if there were more nurses. The complaint is fundamental. The 'tight' staffing levels introduced in an attempt to cut out waste and inefficiency in the NHS have resulted in savings not related to waste or inefficiency. Staff who take maternity leave are not replaced. Replacements are not always made when a member of staff goes off 'sick'. The staff who remain bear the burden for their colleagues. They feel their goodwill and commitment to the NHS is being abused.

While the demands inherent in nursing such as the responsibility for patients' lives and coping with death and dying may cause stress and worry, they are acceptable and not the basis for discontent. It is the externally imposed constraints that cause a lowering of morale. In management terms, it is an inefficient way to run any system. It is a particularly inappropriate way to run a system which is facing a 'demographic time bomb' of too small a pool from which potential recruits into nursing can be drawn.

Nursing is a difficult job at the best of times. The needless imposition of additional stress implies firstly, that the special demands of nursing are not recognized; and, secondly, that the management hierarchy appears to be uncaring about its nurses. It seems likely that this neglect of the nursing workforce is in part due to the gender of the workforce and the perception of nurses as being a disposable and easily replaceable workforce.

It is with indignation that many nurses react to the way that they are being treated. However, there is still a great deal of resistance amongst nurses to actively demonstrating their dissatisfaction with the treatment they are given by the NHS (see Chapter 8). Perhaps nurses have been too passive and quiet in the face of the mounting encroachments on the quality of care they can give.

Notes

1 Menzies (1970), p. 5.
2 West and Rushton (1986), p. 29.
3 See Reid, N.G. (1985a) 'The effective training of nurses: manpower implications', *International Journal of Nursing Studies*, 22:2, p. 94.
4 Menzies (1970), p. 30.
5 See Redfern (1978). For an analysis of the relationship between absence and turnover see Hill, J.M.M. and Trist, E.L. (1962) *Industrial Accidents, Sickness and Other Absences*, London, Tavistock.
6 Also Clark (1975), p. 63.

7 DHSS (1982), p. 26.
8 Violence against nurses appears to be increasing, see Salvage, J. and Rogers, R. (1988) *Nurses at Risk: A Guide to Health and Safety at Work*, London, Heinemann.
9 Some appreciation of the extent of back injuries amongst nurses can be gained from Howie, C. (1987a) 'Back breaking work takes its toll' *The Health Services Journal*, 8 January, 97:5032, pp. 34–5.
10 D. Stubbs at the University of Surrey's Ergonomics Unit cited by Howie ibid. p. 34.
11 DHSS (1972), p. 5.
12 DHSS (1972), p. 39 also reported that many nurses and learners felt they were doing non-nursing work.
13 See Appendix 1 (from the Royal College of Nursing) *in* DHSS (1986) p. 25.
14 Forty-five per cent of the leavers and 39 per cent of stayers reported in the questionnaire that they felt their skills and talents were not being properly used.
15 For an overview of the literature of stress and nursing see Marshall, J. (1980) 'Stress amongst nurses' *in* Cooper, C.L. and Marshall, J. (eds) *White Collar and Professional Stress*, New York, Wiley.
16 Menzies (1970), p. 5.
17 Muir Gray, J.A. (1980) 'Warning: cigarettes may do you good', *Nursing Mirror*, 10 April, p. 22.
18 Contrasts between the stress experienced by general and psychiatric nurses were made by N. Dolan in Northern Ireland, (1987) 'The relationship between burnout and job satisfaction in nurses', *Journal of Advanced Nursing*, 12:1, pp. 3–12.
19 See Merrison (1979), p. 34.
20 Greenborough, J.H. (1985) *Second Report on Nursing Staff, Midwives and Health Visitors* (Review Body for Nursing Staff, Midwives, Health Visitors and Professions Allied to Medicine) London, HMSO, Cmnd. 9529, p. 7.
21 Royal Commission on the National Health Service (1978) *The Working of the National Health Service*, Research Paper No. 1, London, HMSO, p. 5.
22 Revans cited *in* Royal College of Nursing (1978a) *An Assessment of the State of Nursing in the National Health Service*, RCN submission to the Secretary of State for Social Services, London, RCN, p. 43.
23 Davidson (1987), p. 107.
24 Cherniss, C. (1980) *Professional Burnout in Human Service Occupations*, New York, Praeger, p. 5.

6

Hopes and Aspirations: Discrepancies Between Nurses and Employers

Nowhere is it clearer that the aspirations of women working, as nurses, are not being met than in relation to promotion, training and pay. Although a workforce in which career breaks and part-time working are normal, little or no allowance is made to adapt the standard male conditions of employment to the needs of women. The system is geared to the single person working full time with an unbroken career. The demands for childcare facilities, flexible working, training and promotion opportunities for part-time nurses are simply not met. Defences against the failure to provide sufficient training or levels of pay have been built up by nurses: the anti-academic sentiments and the idea of vocation. These defences also combine to ensure that nurses stay quiescent in the face of dissatisfactions. It has perhaps been too easy for managers to ignore the various aspirations of nurses. However, waiting in the wings to pick off those nurses whose needs are not being met are the providers of private health care.

It soon became apparent in conversation with the nurses that their career aspirations were not being met. There was a discrepancy between what the employers were providing and what nurses wanted. Before looking in greater detail at this discrepancy it will be helpful to reiterate some basic information that emerged about these nurses in order to provide the context in which these nurses' hopes and aspirations emerged.

Two-thirds of the nurses were married. Nearly half of the nurses had children. In conversation with the nurses it became obvious that it is normal for their careers in the NHS to be broken. Career breaks are made for a variety of reasons but most are related to having and looking after children. The normality of career breaks in a nurse's working life do not appear to be properly taken into account by managers within the NHS. Similarly, that most nurses are married and many have children appear to be unpalatable facts not properly taken into account by managers within the NHS. Nurses and learners appear to be treated as a disposable, easily replaceable workforce.[1]

Because the questionnaire was addressed towards issues surrounding nurse recruitment and retention, detailed information on the improvements necessary to encourage trained nurses to stay in the NHS was obtained. It is interesting to compare the questionnaire data with the more complex information obtained through the conversations I had with nurses. In the questionnaires pay, predictably, emerged as the single most important improvement. Both for an increase in salary and for special responsibility pay there was resounding enthusiasm. These aspects were rated by nurses to be 'very important' or 'important' by 94 per cent and 80 per cent respectively. It has been argued elsewhere that pay becomes an issue only when other aspects of work become unsatisfactory.[2] However, there was no doubt whatsoever that pay is a real bone of contention amongst many nurses. The situation has, of course, since altered with the 1988 Pay Review Body pay award. Nevertheless, nurses' comments on pay are worth recording. Their attitudes to pay are far from simple.

In conversation I asked the nurses what they thought of their pay. Nearly a quarter thought that their pay was all right.

> Obviously it could be better but it's enough. You can worry too much about the money. (Staff Nurse)

> It's quite good – I'm happy with it. (Sister)

Under a quarter of the nurses said that the pay was all right for *them*, but felt that for others the pay was not good.

> It's adequate if you are a single person, but if you're married and dependent on it . . . (Staff Nurse – who was single)

> . . . for a female like me its all right but for a man with a family it isn't, not when you have kids and mortgage to pay. (Enrolled Nurse)

Over half of the nurses, however, felt that the pay was not good – to put it mildly.

> I think it's atrocious really – it's donkey pay for donkey work. (Student)

. . . it's not worth getting out of bed for (Staff Nurse)

Bloody low considering policemen when they start at almost double what we get. (Staff Nurse)

Disgusting. My Mum's a teacher, she knows how I feel. She doesn't get paid that much either but even she says you could do with a 100 per cent payrise. Then perhaps in a way, even if it was stressful and was hard work, I might be prepared to stick it. (Staff Nurse)

Pay was identified as the single most important aspect of the job which should be improved to encourage trained nurses to stay. Yet a substantial minority of nurses are not complaining about their own pay. On looking closer at the nurses' replies the influence of other factors becomes apparent. First of all, the nurses who say that *their* pay is all right but for others – men, chief breadwinners, single parents – it is not good, are overwhelmingly married women whose husbands are working. While their own reason for working may be economic, the relative amount of their pay is not critical. Because they are married and because they are women they accept more easily the level of salary they are offered. These nurses appear to have accepted some of the attitudes of the wider society to women's employment, i.e. that somehow it is not as worthy as men's employment. Secondly, it is obvious that many of these nurses have a notion of a 'family wage'. In other words, the income for the breadwinner, the head of the family should be enough to support a family. The single, childless person does not need the same amount of money. Thus, some single nurses find their wage all right but have doubts as to how their colleagues manage. A third factor is implicit in many of the 'satisfied' nurses comments: that nursing is a vocation.

I think we should be on more money than what we are but we would not be in the job for money – we have never been well paid have we. What I say is if you want lots of money don't be a nurse. (Patricia)

When we went into nursing we weren't in for the money . . . (Enrolled Nurse)

There are two parts to this notion of vocation. In the first place, people enter nursing because they want to nurse and be 'of service' to others. [3] And in the second place, if the money was to be improved, the 'wrong' sort of person would come into nursing.

Yes I think we're overworked and underpaid but somebody once pointed out that if the wages were very good like the police force, you get the wrong type of people coming into it. You get people coming into it for the money, not because they want to do it. (Laura)

There appears to be a belief within the ranks of nurses that anyone who nursed simply for the money would not be a good nurse. 'I don't really look at it. I mean as long as I've got enough money to get by I don't mind' (Staff Nurse). These nurses may feel unable to complain about their level of pay because it might weaken their own sense of having a vocation. But they *can* complain about the wages of other nurses.

Apart from the ideas of a 'family wage' and of nurses having a vocation, the third major perspective involves a comparison with peers outside the ranks of nursing. Thus, some student nurses may favourably compare themselves with university students on a grant. However, most comparisons are unfavourable. Learners, in particular, make comparisons with the pay they received in other jobs before they started nursing.

I used to be a clerk and I took home £100 a week plus what I could make in bonuses plus free holidays thrown in. The past few months, I've got £52 a week and it's really hard because you get used to a certain lifestyle. (Barbara)

Comparisons are also made with other occupations, in particular with the police.

We have a community policeman. A couple of years ago an 18–20-year-old p.c. came into the unit to see us. And what he said about his salary! I got out my pay slip and he got his pay slip out and he nearly died when he saw how much more he got than I did for the responsibility I was taking. He was just so embarrassed that he earned so much more than I did. (Sister)

I am fairly high up in the management tree and paid less than a police constable. Now that to me is appalling. He's at the bottom of his tree and I am pretty near the top of my tree and I am paid less than he is. (Sister)

The police are the favourite occupation for comparison because nurses see them as performing a similar type of role.

. . . it is similar to the work that the police do in that they work the same shifts and they're dealing with the same sort of things . . . When things go wrong in people's lives it is usually the police or hospitals who see it really . . . (Staff Nurse)

The inordinate difference in pay between the two occupations, therefore, rankles considerably. It is worth noting that a quarter of the learners thought they might join the police once they qualified as nurses. According to Greenborough,[4] comparison of nurses' pay should normally be made with social workers and teachers. However, these occupations are dominated by women and in making comparisons with a female occupation, the disparities between men and women's rates of pay remain unaddressed. At the same time, and perhaps more importantly, nurses themselves very seldom use these two occupational groupings for comparison. It seems that nurses feel they have more in common with their uniformed brothers [*sic*] in the police.

Comparison is also made with work which is less stressful or which requires little training.

. . . the girls in Marks & Spencers get paid more than we do. (Enrolled Nurse)

It really annoys me when . . . My sister-in-law works in a shop where there is no training involved. Fair enough she probably works as hard as I do. But she didn't have to put up with a very low income as a learner for 3 years and you know what kind of status is attached to that. And she takes home more money than I do, which I think is wrong. (Charge Nurse)

Finally, it is worth noting that, on the whole, nursing officers were not dissatisfied with their pay. Most felt that their level of pay was 'better than it's ever been'.

Nursing officers seemed cautious regarding the pay of other grades. There was certainly no general agreement that nurses' pay ought to be improved. The pay of unqualified staff, the nursing assistants and auxiliaries, was mentioned as being low by two nursing officers. Three nursing officers mentioned that pay was a necessary improvement in order to keep and attract trained nurses. Overall from the comments of the nursing officers there was a feeling that expressions of dissatisfaction from less senior nurses about pay would not be sympathetically received. In turn this could be evidence of a lack of contact between some nursing officers and rank-and-file nurses.

According to the questionnaire respondents 'regular training opportunities' was the second most important improvement to keep nurses in the NHS. Most nurses felt that regular training opportunities were 'very important' or 'important'. It is an interest in training which was reflected elsewhere in the questionnaire. The vast majority of nurses would consider doing further training as a nurse. Less than a quarter said they would not consider doing any further training. Half of the nurses had already, at some stage in their career, moved nursing jobs in order to undertake further training. This interest in training is nothing new. In 1972, Briggs reported a high level of interest in further training.[5]

The nurses whom I talked to also showed considerable interest in training. Three-quarters would consider doing further training. Indeed, quite a few of the nurses leaving the Health Authority were going on a course related to nursing. Also, many 'stayers' were about to embark on a course of one type of another. The nurses' interest in doing further training was, however, not always easy to maintain. Many barriers or disincentives to further training were identified.

Getting on a course may be difficult: some courses have waiting lists; Health Authority funds may be limited; and there was competition in securing a place on particularly coveted training courses.

> There's plenty of courses, but there's never enough money to get on, especially things like intensive care and burns. The waiting lists are 5 or 6 years to get on it. (Staff Nurse)

> There is not the money in the Health Service now to allow them [nurses] to keep up to date. We can send one sister and one staff nurse for an update course every year . . . and this leads to a certain amount of rivalry. 'Why has she gone on this course? I've been working here for 8 years and I've never been on a course.' And there are little frictions that go on . . . (Sister)

It may be difficult for a nurse to be spared from her wardwork.

> There are a lot of courses open to qualified nurses, but it's 'if the ward can spare you', you see. I have done one course but the ward wasn't very well covered but I thought I had to do at least one course. (Enrolled Nurse)

Quite understandably, not all courses are offered by each Health Authority. However, for those nurses who have domestic commitments, moving to another area for a few months to do a training course may not be feasible. Similarly, extended further training means a drop in income so those with domestic responsibilities may find it hard to manage.

> I have thought about further training. I wanted to do my RMN [mental nurse training] but once you have a family it is out. I could have done it straight after my training but I already had one child then and I decided not to bother. (Staff Nurse)

Secondment by the Health Authority is by no means automatic. If a nurse leaves the Health Authority to take up a training course on her own, there is no guarantee that a job will be available for her should she wish to return.

Many nurses felt they were not encouraged to undertake further training.

> This course I'm going on, I've had to do everything off my own back. Nobody has encouraged me. I've done everything by myself. (Staff Nurse)

> At present I am happily employed in [another] Health Authority but whilst at [this] Health Authority I found in-service training inadequate, having to pay for evening courses to assist me in my daily occupation. (Staff Nurse)

Enrolled nurses said their training opportunities were very limited in comparison with staff nurses.

> It's all more staff nurse orientated, there's not much for SENs at all. (Enrolled Nurse)

> I'd like to learn a bit more about eyes. At one time we were able to do courses but that's another thing that seems to have been cut back . . . I'm 51 – nursing seems to think I'm too old to learn anything but I'm willing to try. But they are phasing out the enrolled nurse so they are not bothering. (Enrolled Nurse)

Similarly, nurses who work part time do not appear to enjoy the same opportunities for further training as their colleagues:

> Part-time nurses are considered as very much second-class members of the team, given no opportunity or encouragement to embark on further studies or courses. This appears to be management policy. (Staff Nurse)

Finally, there are not always any tangible benefits in undertaking further training.

> I have been very fortunate in that I've had a great deal of training. I've had management courses, industrial relations, all sorts of things, but it hasn't actually altered where I am at the moment. I'm sure if I'd just gone along and perhaps not done middle- or first-line management I would be in exactly the same position as I am now. (Sister)

In a number of areas nurses identified a need for additional training, especially in 'management skills'. Some sisters complained they had been promoted without receiving *any* management training. They had to learn 'on the job' and then, if they were lucky, would receive their first-line management training. (Corroborating comments were also made by nursing officers.)

> When I went on the course – it was designed for newly 'made-up' staff nurses – I'd been a sister for 2 years when I went on it, so I found a lot of the things they were telling me I'd already found out, and found out by making mistakes. I'd learnt the hard way. (Bank Nurse)

Similarly, the lack of management training component within the basic training of staff nurses (who after all are tomorrow's sisters) was also bemoaned.

> Most newly qualified staff nurses will agree that the training they have had does not adequately prepare them to manage the ward alone without placing them under severe stress and anxiety. (Staff Nurse)

Criticisms were also made of the failure to offer refresher courses to nurses who were returning to work after an extended break.

> I think the people who have been out of nursing for a long time would benefit greatly from a 'back-to-nursing' course. A course where they could actually see new techniques, see what's happened while they've been away. (Sister)

There appears to be a half-hearted attitude towards the training of nurses. Obviously there is a *demand* and there is a *need* for further training. As Merrison pointed out a decade ago, 'Basic nursing education can only be a foundation. It needs to be followed by systematic updating and more advanced preparation for specialised roles through post-basic educational programmes'.[6] Perhaps training is seen as an optional extra[7] rather than as a basic necessity in keeping the skills of the nursing workforce up to date and extending those skills. Within the Health Authority there appeared to be variations between the various hospitals and services in the amount of finance available for and the degree of commitment to, further training. Nevertheless, generally there appeared to be what one nursing officer called 'a tight budget' regarding training. However, it was obvious that most nursing officers I talked to were firmly committed to and strongly believed in, the benefits of training.

Nursing officers have to juggle the demands of service and having enough nurses with the need to improve the expertise of their staff. The major influencing factor may be the overall structure and organization of health care rather than influences coming from within the system of nursing. For example, one sister was particularly incensed by the differential treatment of nurses and doctors:

> I think nurses on the whole, especially trained nurses feel very disgruntled with regard to the amount of studying and post-basic training they are allowed compared to say the amount of money that is spent on medical staff. I mean they are allowed to go on study days, study weeks, college conferences and that sort of thing. I think it's very hard for nurses to accept that they can't have a study day to their theatre association congress. They find it very difficult and I think they are very bitter about it. (Sister)

There seems an assumption that once nurses have received their basic training that they need little else to be good nurses. The opposite is true of the medical profession, and should be true of nursing.[8] Newly qualified doctors do not enjoy much status or deference. To obtain that, they first need experience and further knowledge. Indeed, it is accepted that doctors should vigorously pursue the acquisition of further knowledge. To eschew the pursuit of further knowledge would damn the medical profession in the eyes of the public. If further training possibilities for nurses are becoming increasingly limited will this relegate nurses to being second-rate?

There is an interesting and curious distinction between the obvious desire for greater training opportunities within nursing and the widely held distrust of the academically clever nurse (see also Chapter 11). The most convincing explanation focuses on the importance of practical skills in nursing. Thus, it is argued, a 'good' practical nurse does not necessarily need to be highly intellectual. By the same argument, an academically bright person may make a poor bedside nurse. Further training, on the other hand, is given to nurses who have already demonstrated their practical skills and so it does not weaken the belief in the need for such skills. Practical and academic skills are seen as almost mutually exclusive.

This anti-education bias[9] does little service to nurses. While a clever doctor is admired a clever nurse is suspect.[10] The word 'clever' takes on a different connotation in each context. Clever equals bright or intelligent for doctors; but equals smart, cerebral, uncaring for nurses. Perhaps on similar lines was the epithet 'blue stocking' applied to intellectual women in the 1920s! Whatever the origins and basis for the belief, it certainly enables others to underestimate the demands which nursing makes. It must affect the level of self-esteem that nurses have for their own skills and capabilities, and for those of their colleagues. Thus, the approval of doctors rather than nurses may be sought.[11] Denying the need for nurses to be clever, certainly does not raise the status or prestige of nurses amongst non-nursing colleagues. The anti-academic sentiment also can act so as to reduce dissatisfaction with the lack of training opportunities, just as the notion of vocation acts to limit the demands for greater levels of pay.

Given the numerous barriers and difficulties facing nurses wanting further training, it is surprising that there is still such a level of interest. Some of this interest may be a reflection of the need of nurses to get out of the clinical environment for a while if the pressures are felt to be too great. And it must not be forgotten that an interest in training often disguises an interest in promotion. Further training in another Health Authority may also involve an offer of a permanent job. In other words, interest in further training may be another manifestation of the movement encouraged by the systems surrounding nursing.[12] It could well be that many nurses are 'late developers' who become interested in realizing their own potential only once they have achieved a level of expertise and confidence. Dex, for example, found a sizeable under-achievement amongst women as they left school.[13] Training within nursing may offer such women a second chance at realizing their own potential. However, it should not be forgotten that some recruits to nursing are academically very well qualified and further nurse training has always been on their agenda.

A third improvement which the nurses completing the questionnaire felt necessary to keep trained nurses in the NHS was 'better promotion possibilities'. Thus, 85 per cent felt that 'better promotion possibilities' were 'important' or 'very important' in retaining qualified staff. Not many nurses are happy with their promotion prospects, at least to judge from the stayers responses. (The leavers were not asked about this aspect in the questionnaire.) Well over half felt their promotion prospects were either 'not very good' or 'poor' while only a quarter felt they were 'quite good'. (The rest were unsure about their promotion prospects.) In comparison with the findings of Briggs in 1972, promotion prospects appear to have worsened.[14,15] For the leavers a 'lack of promotion prospects' was the second most often given reason for leaving. (The most frequently given reason was to have a baby.) Thus, in order to obtain promotion, many nurses had to move to another hospital or Health Authority. Poor promotion prospects are undoubtedly a real problem for many nurses. The lack of promotion prospects are most keenly felt in three areas. Firstly, part-time staff are seldom considered for promotion: 'Promotion is virtually non-existent as a part-time member of staff. Your years of experience are not taken into consideration at all' (Sister). Secondly, there are too few opportunities for promotion from staff nurse level.

I don't think I'd want to do anything else now. The only thing that is missing for me now is career development. Just to be able to get to a charge nurse and to actually be in charge of somewhere, work and put your own ideas forward. Stamp your individuality on something. Well . . . possibly 5 years ago it would have been easy for me to get a charge nurse, but it's nearly impossible now. (Staff Nurse)

I've been a staff nurse for $5\frac{1}{2}$ years. Now some people might say that's not very long but I had hoped to achieve more than I have in the last 5 years . . . I've had to move and travel to get my [promotion to sister] . . . (Staff Nurse)

Thirdly, sisters and charge nurses who want to remain clinically involved are unable to take promotion because it means moving into management.

I don't want to go any further, I am quite happy as I am. I don't want a lot of paperwork. I would rather be on the other end of it, doing the work. (Sister)

I don't want to go into management. I came into nursing to be involved with people . . . I think perhaps if I had a nursing officer's job 5–7 years ago it was a totally different matter, I could have quite enjoyed that. But not the present type of management. (Charge Nurse)

The unwillingness to move out of the clinical area does mean less competition and frustration for those who seek promotion. And there is always a need for highly experienced nurses at sister/charge nurse level. Yet there is some evidence of frustration amongst this level of nurse because they can become stale in their jobs. However, there are other options open to the highly experienced nurse. One avenue is to move into community nursing as a health visitor and many sisters and the occasional charge nurse do so. However, blockages occur within the community nursing service as in any speciality.

What on earth the district will do when we all retire I shudder to think, I really do, because there are so many of us who are are 40s/early 50s and above. There's a few young ones coming on but not that many . . . With so many of us being in post there is not the jobs for the younger ones, if they wanted to go on the district. (District Nurse)

One of the reasons given for the 'blockages' in the promotion prospects of the hospital-based nurses was the increased use of maternity leave.

> . . . there used to be quite a turnover whereas people now are
> hanging on. Whereas some of them who left maternity-wise are
> hanging on to their jobs now, which you can't blame them, if
> they need to . . . And talking to friends from other hospitals, it's
> just the same there, very little promotion. (Male Staff Nurse)

There is no sign that frustrations with the lack of promotion prospects
are going to diminish. On the contrary, the removal of a number of
nursing officer posts means even further restrictions on promotion.
With such limited promotion opportunities it is not surprising that
promotion is sometimes used as a stick to ensure 'good behaviour'.
Thus one nurse having had a tussle with the Director of Nursing
Services which also involved her nursing officer was told that 'she had
really made a mess for herself'. Essentially the nurse felt she was being
told that if she pursued the matter she would not be considered for
promotion.

The present career structure of nurses does not offer many
opportunities for promotion. This, however, is in the process of
changing with the acceptance of a new grading structure allied to the
pay increases given in April 1988.

What the outcome of these changes in grade structures will be is
open to conjecture as is their reception by the nursing profession. For
the moment, promotion is not felt to be a problem within the Health
Service. However, promotion is not felt to be a problem by all nurses.
Learners are too busy trying to become qualified to be much
concerned with promotion – the dizzy heights of staff nurse are
sufficiently high for them at the moment. The enrolled nurse grade
has traditionally not been a career grade and many enrolled nurses
are happy with their bedside nursing role. Indeed, less than half of
them said they would be seeking to go on a conversion course to
become a registered nurse. A few enrolled nurses are not content with
their very limited promotion prospects but they appear to be the
exception. Thus, one enrolled nurse said that a recently opened
private hospital was trying to capitalize on the proposed phasing out
of the enrolled nurse grade:

> . . . the enrolled nurses, if they don't want to do the bridging
> course, have got the opportunity of becoming senior enrolled
> nurses, which is promotion. It's the same as a staff nurse. That's
> how they are luring them with the prospects of promotion,
> whereas here there is no chance even for a staff nurse for
> promotion. (Enrolled Nurse)

Like some enrolled nurses, many part-time nurses were often happy to undertake fairly undemanding work as they devoted the bulk of their time and energy to their families. Nevertheless, the period spent doing part-time work is really time spent in the wilderness because it means that a nurse's career is put into abeyance. It also means that maximum use is not made of nurses' skills. Using ex-ward sisters as bank nurses who are shunted onto a different ward each night whose routine, patients, and procedures are unfamiliar solves a short-term problem. However, it was quite apparent that some of these bank nurses had minimal involvement in their work which they did not like.

> I've switched off. That's why I just go and do the work and that's it. I do nights mostly so its not the same sort of situation as it is during the day. I just get on with the work that I'm used to doing . . . I did apply for a full-time post as a night sister but I wasn't even short listed. I was a ward sister for 5 years but presumably I've been out of it too long. (Bank Nurse)

By taking up bank nursing the return to nursing after a break may become easier.[16] However, as Salvage argues, nurses may be forced into working on the bank because their needs for childcare facilities, flexible hours, part-time work, etc. are not being met by the NHS.[17] The difficulty of 'getting back into' nursing was often mentioned.

> I was a theatre sister before I had the children but it is very hard to get back in on nights . . . I would like to go back to Theatre eventually but the longer you are out of it the more difficult it is to get back in. (Bank Nurse)

And even when a nurse does manage to get back in to permanent employment, it may be necessary to accept demotion if what you want is part-time work. In turn this presents difficulties for nurses who are used to being in charge.

> I think particularly that part-time staff nurses have got no say. Once when I'd just come back to nursing I said I'd phoned the doctor because nobody had been to see his patient and I really got in trouble because they said: 'Oh you should see the night sister, she has to decide whether you ring the doctor'. Well having been used to just picking up the phone and ringing for a doctor when I wanted to speak to a doctor that just did it. I was ticked off for using my initiative and brains. (Bank Nurse – ex Sister)

Quite a number of nurses found it difficult to combine the roles of nurse and parent.

Really I don't think full-time nursing and a family go together –
you can't give to both the same. (Bank Nurse)

I feel that for most women eventually a choice has to be made –
career or home life. It is impossible to remain as a part-time
nursing sister in one specialty. Part-time staff tend to be moved
to different areas. (Staff Nurse)

Having to make such a choice is not easy particularly for first-time
parents who do not know how they will cope with a young child. The
impact of a young child can be quite dramatic and unexpected:

I don't resent having him [her baby son] but I never realized how
much it could interfere with your life really. I thought I could just
carry on and go back when I wanted and it would all fit in nicely
and that, but it's not that easy. I think if you weren't bothered
about doing things properly it would be easier but if you want to
look after him well and do your job well, it's hard isn't it? (Staff
Nurse)

Many nurses were well aware of the difficulties they might encounter
with a young child: problems with child-minding being the most
prominent. 'I didn't take maternity leave because I have a problem
with getting somebody to mind the baby . . . (Sister). A few nurses
who were leaving because they were pregnant were planning to
return full time (in order to fulfil their maternity leave requirements)
and later take part-time work. Only a few were going to try to
continue in full-time employment, often for financial reasons:

At the moment we can't really afford for me to drop. (Sister)

I think I will have to financially. I don't know that I really want
to. (Sister)

Others had decided to leave nursing completely – at least for the time
being. 'Obviously the baby is more important than the job' (Staff
Nurse).

This Health Authority offered no crèche or nursery facilities. Yet
over three-quarters of the nurses who completed a questionnaire felt
the provision of crèche facilities was 'important' or 'very important' in
keeping trained nurses.

Hospital crèches are *very* important as many mothers like me,
without family nearby, are loathe to leave children with child-
minders. (Staff Nurse)

All nursing jobs are important – many part-timers would work
full-time if crèches were available. (Staff Nurse)

The need for crèche facilities was raised by many nurses whom I spoke to. The more senior nurses said how good it would have been for them if there had been crèche facilities:

> At a hospital where I used to work they had a crèche facility and the girls found that very satisfactory because they could go and give the children their lunch and they were within calling distance and they knew they were in a controlled environment whereas the child-minders – you've got no idea of what they are going to do, its always at the back of your mind. (Sister)

> In the earlier days a crèche would have been very useful, but now the children are of school age its more difficult to be reasonable to expect them to do it. (Charge Nurse)

The more junior nurses emphasized the benefits that a crèche would bring them today. Thus, a staff nurse who has applied to return to full-time working said:

> A crèche would be super – it would be the end of all my problems. They don't make it easy for women with very small children. Although I worked part time you've still got to be there for half past seven in the morning and my husband leaves at quarter to seven so . . . it was just very difficult. (Staff Nurse)

It was emphasized in a variety of ways that crèches make it possible for nurses to stay on at work despite having young children. Crèches, it was argued, could increase the number of nurses who could work full time rather than part time. Many parents worried about their children if they are looked after by child-minders. Obviously if Health Authorities wish to retain their qualified staff (or any female staff) they will have to start providing crèche facilities.

> If they had a crèche in the hospitals of the future I'm sure that would help tremendously [to keep nurses] – it really would. (Sister)

> Crèche facilities would be a good idea because a lot of people leave because of the children, there's no one to look after them. And by the time they've paid to have a child-minder it's not worth working at all. (Sister)

Some years ago when nurses were not in great supply, accommodation to the needs of their female workforce was obviously necessary.

> It's something that has actually gone full circle because when I went back after I had my children, there was much more freedom about hours that you worked. Now you can't: you either work

full time or you work on the bank virtually. Whereas I was given an awful lot of choice about hours: 'well what would you like to work' sort of thing. You know, I think we have to become more flexible about the hours the nurses work and try and fit in better with one another's commitments. (Sister)

There have been a number of social changes in the last two or three decades. Many more women go back to work after they have had children. There has been a large increase in the number of women working in part-time jobs. There is no evidence that women actually prefer part-time work – it is simply that part-time work for women is increasingly available.[18] At the same time there has been a large increase in the divorce rate. Many marriages break down. Women who have been quite happily working part or full time find that when their marriage breaks up they are unable to continue working. Similarly, problems can be caused by a non-cooperating ex-spouse.

I don't want to leave nights. I'm divorced and my daughter goes to her Dad's at the weekend while I'm working. He won't have her any more and so I've been forced to get on to days, which . . . for her it's good because I will see more of her and I will have my weekends free. I've got to go to a child-minder – it's going to cost me £18 more so I'm going to be worse off because I lose my night allowance. (Enrolled Nurse)

Not only do women bear the children they also bear the brunt of caring for the children. There were not many cases of role reversal, where the husband stayed at home with the children, amongst these nurses. However, it was apparent that many spouses tried to share the burdens (and rewards) of childcare and housework.[19]

They [the children] are both of school age and my wife works set days. I manage to sort out my days so that one week we are fine, I'm there. The rest of the time they are either at school, my wife drops them off before she goes to work, and I finish early or some-one else brings them home, so we manage – but it is a problem. (Charge Nurse)

Many nurses do manage to combine successfully work with their young children. Often there are financial reasons but, also for many, staying at home is difficult after they have become accustomed to a demanding and fulfilling job.

I had no intention of staying away for good. I was anxious to get back – financial reasons and boredom really. I'm not the type to stay at home all the time. (Staff Nurse)

I was pregnant and fully intended to leave until the children went to school but I just found I needed to do some work. It wasn't purely for financial reasons. I mean obviously it helped but I needed something outside the home. (Health Visitor)

Another bone of contention for many nurses is the failure for working hours to reflect in any way to the fact that nurses are frequently parents. A greater provision of flexible working hours was mentioned by well over half of the nurses as being 'important' or 'very important' in retaining qualified nurses in the NHS. The difficulties faced by those with children is also reflected in the finding that a quarter of the questionnaire nurses said that having to look after children might cause them to leave nursing. Over a third said that having a baby might cause them to leave nursing. To reduce the possibility of nurses leaving the Health Service in the future flexible working hours and the provision of child care facilities will have to be addressed. When the shortage of nurses really starts to bite, things might have to change.

In conversation with nurses it became obvious that it is fairly normal for their careers in the NHS to be broken. Career breaks are made for a variety of reasons but most are related to having and looking after children. The demands of a partner or spouse also have a role to play in career breaks. Fitting in with a partner's hours of work and holidays, moving to another area. While many other factors such as dependent relatives, a nurse's own health, change of religion (surprisingly frequently mentioned) may be influential, none compare to the impact of children or partner on nurses' career patterns.

These career breaks vary considerably in length. Some last for a few months, others for 20 years. The length of career break is not necessarily planned. Nurses may envisage staying at home with their children until they reach school age. But once at home, boredom or frustration at being 'out of things' often occurs. Quite a number of nurses mentioned that they found they were not the type to stay at home. ' . . . it wasn't purely from financial reasons. I mean obviously it helped but I needed something outside the home' (Staff Nurse).

There appeared to be an acceptance amongst quite a few of the nurses who were mothers that they *ought* to stay at home and be with their children. Yet, the hustle and bustle of everyday nursing was missed. There was also a suggestion that these women, who often had a great deal of responsibility at work, felt under-used at home. The popular belief held by quite a number of nurses that a women's place is in the home was displaced by the demands and rewards of nursing. 'I missed my nursing' (Enrolled Nurse).

The importance of a career to many nurses was quite apparent. But the main reason for returning to nursing is money (see Appendix 8), while being able to leave the family is also important. The decision to return to nursing is not always an easy one:

> I must admit I did hum and haw about whether I wanted to go back into nursing although I'd always enjoyed it, mainly because having now got children I wasn't sure how I could cope with looking after a family and a very demanding job. (Sister)

Nurses who were leavers had proportionately more breaks in their career than stayers. One possible explanation for this is the greater number of nurses choosing or needing to return to work when they have younger children, than say 10–15 years ago. Unemployment continues to be fairly high in the area and even although only a few nurses had a partner who was unemployed the previous unemployment of partners was quite often mentioned. The primary reason for returning to work – money – lends support to this explanation. Similarly, many nurses spoke of their partner being made redundant and of the threat of redundancy. Economic factors were obviously influential in these nurses' career decisions.

Yet leavers less often identified money, childcare, or 'wanting to get out of the house' as influential reasons in returning to nursing. It may be that one response to constraints is to simply take them for granted. In other words, when you are out of nursing in order to look after children and with little chance of being able to return to work, the perceived influence of factors such as money is weaker.[20] Many nurses who leave to look after their children have every intention of returning to nursing, whether on a part-time or full-time basis. Of the nine pregnant nurses who were 'leavers', only three were not taking maternity leave. These three were unsure as to whether or not they would go back to nursing in the short or the longer term. The other six pregnant nurses said they intended to return to full-time working. Three of these were intending to transfer to part-time work after they had completed the requisite full-time stint – if they had the choice. It is worth noting here that the option of part-work is not open to many senior nurses – they must return to full-time working.

Breaks have always been interpreted negatively. For the NHS it means losing a trained worker and all the bother of replacement. For the individual nurse, breaks in employment mean losing out regarding length of experience, and by extension, promotion. But breaks may also be beneficial to both NHS and the individual nurse. Few dispute that nursing is stressful work. By taking breaks from such work, 'burnout' or overstress may be avoided.[21] Just as withdrawal from work can be a response to stress, so breaks may lengthen the working life of a nurse enabling her/him to temporarily leave nursing and return when under less strain. In other words, nurses may have a shorter career in nursing if they do not have breaks. It has been argued elsewhere that child-bearing interrupts rather than terminates women's working lives.[22] It is up to those within senior nurse management to ensure that women who are nurses, when they return to work, return to nursing. And, to make sure, at the same time, that the career interruptions do not become career terminations.

Those who manage the nursing workforce do not appear, judging by their lack of action, to have actively assisted women who wish to return to nursing. There is some distrust amongst senior nurses regarding the young married (and potentially fertile) women.

Indeed, as with many employers, there is some discrimination against married women within the NHS. It is much easier and simpler to employ single people: they are much less likely to take maternity leave; they are less likely to have to balance demands of children and job; and they are more able to work the various shifts demanded of nurses. Yet single people are just as likely to have dependent relatives to look after and they are often more mobile and more likely to change jobs than their colleagues who have spouses.

Being defined as 'single' is no guarantee that the person has no partner. But the handle of 'married' is likely to affect young women in particular. Young, married women are fairly likely to become pregnant – they are not seen as such a 'safe' bet as older or single women. A nursing officer said she tried not to let marital status affect her judgement when she was interviewing, but:

> I think if we were all honest with ourselves we would say, yes, you would look at the one who is not going to give you as many problems – although it's happened to me that the single one has been the one who has had the most problems – but I think it's very difficult if you are interviewing and you know there is a woman there with a 15-month-old baby and one at school, you begin to think: how well is she going to be coping?

There are very few single women in the senior nursing posts now. Only one nursing officer was single. While they may not have forgotten what it is like to be a parent, the demands of their managerial job, especially that of keeping the unit staffed, is their most pressing problem. It may be that the 'tight' staffing levels ensure that nursing officers cannot empathize too much with their own nurses.

Yet if the NHS does not wake up to the demands of its workforce then the private sector might reap the benefits. 'But I do hope to come back to do some sort of part-time hours. If not here, then some kind of nursing somewhere' (Sister).

The attractions of the private sector were mentioned on a number of occasions. The fact that a new private hospital was headhunting for particular specialist nurses was mentioned often. Feelings regarding the private health care sector are extremely mixed. Nevertheless there is a substantial minority of nurses ready and quite willing to move into the private sector (see also Chapter 11).

It is interesting that the learners were much less antagonistic to private health care than qualified nurses. For example, only one pupil would not consider working in the private sector. The others were generally undecided. It may be that loyalty to the NHS grows as learners progress through their training. However, given the numerous complaints which many nurses have of the NHS now, loyalty to the NHS may be harder and harder to maintain. If the health service becomes less and less something of which nurses can be proud, their loyalty and commitment to it may wear thin. If the private sector can meet the needs of a mainly female workforce by offering, for example, flexible hours they may well find quite a queue of NHS nurses waiting to join them.

Women working part time appear to experience downward mobility in many occupations.[23] However, the acceptance of downward mobility in an occupation which is so overwhelmingly composed of women is lamentable. The failures of the NHS generally to meet the needs of its female workforce have been commented on many times.[24] There has been a particular failure throughout the NHS (with some notable exceptions, such as that by the Welsh Office[25]) to make efforts to offer greater part-time opportunities, etc. for nurses.[26] Present policies play into the hands of the government and its encouragement of the private health-care sector where greater advantage may be taken of the opportunity to acquire nursing staff.

The failure to provide better opportunities for parents to return to nursing may not have been a conspiracy to keep nurses in their place, but it has had that effect. The costs of the disinterest in, and neglect of, the primarily female workforce, are currently being realized in many parts of the country. Shortages of nurses are increasing.[27] The disposable workforce ethos – use-once-and-throw-away – is demeaning to the women who choose to take up nursing as a career. It also serves to reduce the prestige and status of nurses, nursing, and women. Thus, nursing can easily be seen as a job at which women are only playing. At the same time, the work of nurses can be trivialized if it can be done by a perpetual stream of young learners. How, then, can nursing be viewed as having a real contribution to make to the improvement of the health of patients? The past ease of replacement has meant that attempts to develop the skills and potential of the workforce are not made. What a waste!

Notes

1 The UKCC has referred to nurse education as working on a 'constant replacement system' – UKCC (1986), p. 11.
2 See Cherniss (1980), p. 12; Annandale-Steiner, D. (1979) 'Unhappiness is the nurse who expected more', *Nursing Mirror*, 29 November, p. 35.
3 For an introduction to issues surrounding occupational choice see Roberts, K. (1975) 'The developmental theory of occupational choice: a critique and an alternative' *in* Esland, G., Salaman, G., and Speakman, M-A. (eds) *People and Work*, Edinburgh, Holmes McDougall.
4 Greenborough (1985), p. 61.
5 DHSS (1972), p. 72.
6 Merrison (1979), p. 203.
7 Schofield, M. (1986) 'Manpower and personnel policies: the district perspective', *Hospital and Health Services Review*, September, 82:5, p. 206.
8 See Merrison (1979), p. 203.
9 Salvage (1985), p. 77.
10 Bradshaw, P.L. (1984) 'A quaint philosophy', *Senior Nurse*, 28 November, 1:35, p. 11.
11 See Kalisch and Kalisch (1977), p. 53.
12 This has been described as 'officially sponsored touristry' see Pape, R. (1978) *in* Dingwall and McIntosh (eds) Chapter 4; see also Melia (1984), p. 148.
13 Dex, S. (1987) *Women's Occupational Mobility: a Lifetime Perspective*, London, Macmillan, p. 60.
14 DHSS (1972), Chapter 6.
15 The implementation of the Salmon and Griffiths recommendations have had a role to play here – see Carpenter *in* Dingwall and McIntosh (eds) (1978); See Cousins (1987), p. 167.
16 DHSS (1982), p. 22.
17 Salvage (1985), p. 43.
18 For an analysis of the position of women in the labour market, see Walby, S. (1987) *Flexibility and the Changing Sexual Division of Labour*, University of Lancaster, Lancaster Regionalism Group Working Paper 36, p. 14.
19 The burden of housework is not equally shared. Pahl, for example, reports that his data showed 'that women do most of the work in and around the household, even if they are also in employment'. Pahl, R.E. (1984) *Divisions of Labour*, Oxford, Blackwell, p. 327.
20 The reasons for taking a job are not necessarily the same as those for staying, or for leaving, see Goldthorpe J., Lockwood, D., Bechhofer, F. and Platt, J. (1968) *The Affluent Worker: Industrial Attitudes and Behaviour*, Cambridge, CUP and the rejoinder by W.W. Daniel (1969) 'Industrial

behaviour and orientation to work – a critique', *Journal of Management Studies*, 6, pp. 366–75.

21 For definitions of 'burnout' see Lombardi (1987), p. 8; Cherniss (1980), pp. 5–6.

22 Joshi, H. (1984) *Women's Participation in Paid Work: Further Analysis of the Women and Employment Survey*, London, Department of Employment, Research Paper No. 45, p. 47.

23 Dex, S. (1985) *The Sexual Division of Work*, Brighton, Harvest Press, p. 8.

24 DHSS (1972), p. 184; Gaze (1987), p. 25; Hyams, J. (1987) 'Nice nurse: shame about the status', *Company*, July, p. 84.

25 See Department of Health and Social Security (1986b) *Control of Nursing Manpower* (Fourteenth Report from the Committee of Public Accounts Session 1985–6), London, HMSO, p. vi.

26 Merrison (1979), p. 170; Brookes, Long and Rathwell (1987), p. 11; RCN (1987), p. 11.

27 See, for example, RCN (1987).

7

Bitchiness

A particularly keenly felt aspect of nursing is the 'bitchiness'. A lack of support from colleagues, failures of communication together with a system which is unsympathetic to the problems of individuals combine to produce an over-critical working atmosphere. The links made between women working together and the bitchy atmosphere give support to the argument that many nurses have adopted misogynistic attitudes. The increasing demands made on all grades of nurses from staffing levels act to increase the pressures and therefore the unsupportive atmosphere. Speaking-out is frowned upon and the subservient attitudes inculcated during training mean that the muttering about discontents becomes the norm. Once again, the issue of gender emerges as a powerful explanatory factor of what goes on within nursing.

As was shown in the previous chapter, nurses speak of many dissatisfactions in their work. There is a general feeling that little or nothing has been done in the recent past to tackle these areas of dissatisfaction. It is little wonder, therefore, that morale was not felt to be high. Most of the nurses I spoke to felt that morale was not good amongst nurses, particularly, in the large and impersonal general hospital (see Chapter 5). 'The hospital's only drawback is that it's so big – it makes it impersonal really, whereas in these little old hospitals everybody knows each other' (Staff Nurse). Particular units or specialties tended to be self-contained and there seems to be little opportunity to meet staff from other areas.

> I've worked here for $3\frac{1}{2}$ years and I don't know many people here at all and it's not that I never go out of the unit, because if we transfer a patient you try and go upstairs. I might know the odd

> person but I couldn't walk up the corridor and expect to see
> someone I knew. (Staff Nurse)

The anonymity of the large hospital together with the generally low
state of nurse morale was reflected in the way in which nurses relate
to one another. In all the hospitals and specialties it was said again
and again that nurses need to learn to care for each other. Nurses are
frequently felt not to give any support to their colleagues. There also
seems to be a lack of trust between the different grades of nurses.
Indeed, it may have affected the level of response to the questionnaire:

> Because of the lack of trust between nurses on the wards and the
> 'higher ranks' I imagine many people will treat your question-
> naire with great suspicion despite your attempts at reassurance.
> Talking to people they are totally unconvinced that this will not
> get back to the powers that be. (Staff Nurse)

> Some nurses are afraid of the consequences – fear of manage-
> ment in NHS – and will not be sending in these forms. (Sister)

In essence many nurses feel that nurses are bitchy to one another.
This is not a new problem in nursing. From the unsolicited letters
received by the Briggs committee, 'the single greatest cause of
complaint was the attitudes and behaviour of nurses themselves . . .'.[1] The need for care between nurses, and the lack of such care,
has been commented on by others.[2]

Part of the reason for the 'bitchiness' may be that as nurses spend so
much of their compassion on patients that they have little left over for
each other. The strain of smiling to patients who are difficult, to
patients who are dying, to patients who are less than appreciative
may well be reflected in nurses' dealings with one another. Having
constantly to guard your tongue in front of patients may mean that
colleagues bear the brunt of any stress.

> I suppose it's all the time you are working with patients you are
> getting insulted, not insulted but they are nasty to you and they
> say nasty things like 'nobody's bothered about me' – I know a lot
> of them are justified – when there are only three of you looking
> after thirty patients, somebody is going to have to wait. (Sister)

Bitchiness is THE aspect which learners loathe above all else. When
the students and the pupils are asked about their moans after a bad
day, it is problems with other staff which overwhelmingly
predominates.

> If I had a bad day, I'd probably be complaining about the staff.
> Probably no one would care what was wrong with me. I mean

sometimes you want to be asked 'how are you getting on, is there anything bothering you?'. (Eileen)

Probably somebody saying something that has really got me hurt or annoyed or just being expected to do things that you just can't do and they thought you were stupid. (Ann)

Some of the learners were obviously disappointed with the behaviour of nurses to one another.

I don't think people have been as friendly as I thought they might have been. They are friendly but they are not as protective as I would have thought they would be. Sometimes I've seen people being told off for doing something the first time . . . (Barbara)

It is not just new recruits, but all grades of nurses who find the other staff can add to their difficulties.

They [nurses] weren't the kind of professionals that I thought they were. I love the patients. Its just the hassle of the other people and the vibes and all the other staff shouting at each other and shouting at me. (Student)

An explanation often given for the 'bitchiness' in nursing is the fairly frequently aired view that it's due to there being so many women in nursing 'I think it's the same wherever you get a group of women, isn't it really, you're going to get that' (Sally). This explanation was rejected by quite a few nurses, some of whom felt that men were just as bad while others pointed out that the atmosphere on wards varied considerably. 'It's not because it's all women – I think that's a silly thing because women aren't bitchy. Some wards are worse than others, some are just terrible' (Paula). A frequently given reason for the bitchiness was the workload and level of stress under which nurses were working.

I think people just get so overtired and irritable. I mean if it's not direct pressure or stress it's indirect, it's all different ways you can feel it. (Pupil)

I think half of it is the stress and all the women together. And all the cutbacks, I think, that doesn't help and the shortage of staff. You go on in a morning and you just can't see an end; there isn't an end. There's not very many days when I've come back and felt I've done everything I could have done that day. (Student)

Particular specialties have particular difficulties and tensions which are inherent in the work they do.

They are a good crowd of girls but there's a tremendous bitchiness with working in a close-knit environment. It's been in every theatre I've ever worked in. Rivalry? I don't know. Women working closely together? I've never really pinned it down. It's always there in an operating theatre environment. I sometimes wonder if it's to do with the nature of the work. You are suddenly pumping adrenalin into the system, you get an aneurism coming in and there's this great high that you go up and then you come down with a bang when it's all over and . . . your whole day is spent on these highs and lows and I think perhaps that leads to a certain amount of friction. (Sister)

Friction was often reported to exist between those on night and day duty. Complaints about work left undone by the other shift and failure to communicate were mentioned.

It's like the North–South divide between night and day staff . . . Like somebody said the other night they tend to think the night staff are second-class citizens. I think you get it on all the wards, but it's not a permanent thing, it comes and goes. (Staff Nurse)

A lot of nurses are bitchy, especially day and night staff about each other. I suppose they all think their way is best. I think the system between the two of passing messages on leaves something to be desired. Both think the other is totally incompetent. (Alice)

The grumbling atmosphere and the bitchiness are closely allied in the often made comment that nurses feel they lack support. It is not always clear what 'support' means to different nurses. At one level, lack of support means that nurses are not supported in the decisions they take. Thus, one sister said that her main moan about work:

. . . would be the pressure of work and the lack of support for what you decided to do. You know, you can work away all day and know that the following day you may well get harangued for what you've done . . . You come home and you feel that you are constantly battling against a brick wall; that no matter what you do, it isn't going to have been the right thing to have done. (Sister)

If I started moaning it would probably be about the management because you don't get any support for anything and people are just coming back and saying you should have done this, that and the other, and you think well if you could have been here at the time, see what you would have done. (Staff Nurse)

The importance of this felt lack of support should not be underestimated, it may cause nurses to leave: 'Lack of support from higher management for nursing decisions leads to nurses leaving the profession' (Staff Nurse). Other nurses felt that support was lacking from senior nurses who did not look after, or were not interested in, the welfare of nurses.

> It seems that staff reductions and cutbacks are responsible for the don't care attitude of the so-called caring profession towards their own workers. The welfare of the nursing staff seems to be an unimportant issue now. (Staff Nurse)

For many nurses, the failure to formally monitor the health of nurses indicates a lack of care and interest in the nursing workforce.

> Well, we are in a stressful occupation, our backs can get hurt and all that sort of thing, and we're never monitored – we just look after ourselves. All right, everybody else does, but somehow I feel a little bit dissatisfied about that. I think we could have a bit better care taken of us. (District Nurse)

Many nurses complained about not being told what was going on. The need to improve communications was one of the aspects most frequently mentioned in the questionnaires as 'the main thing which should be improved by managers'. Indeed, it was second in importance only to staffing levels for the leavers. There were repeated comments about the failure of communication by senior management and others.

> I think that it might help matters if people were actually told, not just given a memo that this is what is planned, but that people are actually told, sat down with and talked to about it, what the plans are for the NHS and how it will eventually affect them. You know support counts for a great deal and I feel sometimes in the NHS, you don't get it. (Staff Nurse)

Within their own unit most nurses felt they did know 'what was going on'. However, within the hospital or service as a whole, and within the Health Authority itself, the majority felt there was a lack of information. At a time in the Health Service when so much is in the process of being changed, this failure to communicate effectively may be critical. Although Peach can comment that 'in an organisation as huge as the NHS, word of mouth is an important supplement or substitute for paper',[3] this ignores the results of inadequate formal communication. Gossip and rumours take on real significance. Issues get blown up out of all proportion to their importance. And, as the staff nurse above points out, information on paper is not as welcome as personal contact with the decision-maker. The uncertainty of knowledge acquired through rumour is reflected in a further lowering of morale. Information is power; lack of information is evidence of powerlessness. If you are not told what is going on, you may conclude that you are not deemed of sufficient importance to be told.

For many nurses information was limited to what was going on in their own unit of specialty: 'I know what's going on in the unit but I don't know what's going on in the rest of the hospital' (Staff Nurse). Communication is a particular problem with geographically scattered units, shift working and those who work in relative isolation from colleagues, as in community nursing.[4] Each link in the chain of command is important to good communication. Thus, what and how information is passed on by nursing officers and sisters affects what and how information is received. Failures at one level influence attempts to give sufficient information elsewhere.

The failure to communicate reflects poor management skills or disinterest in letting nurses know what is going on. However, if management does not keep nurses informed, there is no reason why they should keep nurses' goodwill. It may be that more and more resistance to change will be encountered amongst nurses for this very reason.

Communication, of course, is a two-way process. Failures of communication also occur when those higher up in the hierarchy get out of touch with those who provide the service.[5] The reduction in the number of nursing officers may well increase the number of failures of communication as nursing officers have less and less time to 'walk the job'.

As it was, senior nurses were often felt not to appreciate the efforts of their nursing staff. It is obvious that many nurses work longer hours than they are required to. At the same time many nurses do their utmost to turn up for work. They dislike going off sick yet if they do feel under the weather at work no one notices or suggests they go home. It seems that staffing levels are so tight that interest in nurses' own welfare is supplanted by the more pressing need to keep the wards or unit running.

> . . .you've got to be practically moribund before they send you home and once you are there that's it. I don't feel anybody cares for us. Nobody. You are just there to do your job, get on with it, no matter what you feel like. (Sister)

> Nobody sort of asks the nurse how she feels, or when did she have a break or whatever. You are just expected to sort of carry on. I think a lot of nurses feel you are just a number; you are just a pair of hands, a pair of feet – get on with it. (Student)

The lack of support and interest by senior nurses is felt to be relatively new. It is the comparison with how things used to be that makes it particularly difficult for some nurses to get used to the less sympathetic climate.

> At one time if nursing staff had any problems which could affect your nursing, you could go to the relevant senior staff and they would try to help or give you consideration in your work, e.g. make sure that you were working with another qualified staff ensuring that all the ward's responsibility is not yours. Now it seems that there is no interest in staff with problems (and we all have problems sometime or other). (Enrolled Nurse)

The operating difficulties of senior nurses appear to overcome any sympathy they might feel for the pressures exerted on their nurses by the heavy workload and the tight staffing levels.

> You can be dying and nobody will say to you: 'Oh go home' or if you ring in sick you are made to feel guilty about ringing in sick. There's a sort of frosty voice saying: 'Oh, what's wrong with you?'. (Enrolled Nurse)

As was shown in Chapter 5 the majority of nurses feel absenteeism is a problem. When staffing levels are already low it causes extra pressure to be put on those who remain at work. As a result many nurses feel resentful when colleagues do not turn up for work. The problem for nurses who are genuinely sick is that they are likely not to be believed when they *are* genuinely sick. Many nurses feel that colleagues do go absent for non-medical reasons. However, the high levels of stress which nurses experience can become as intolerable as a physical illness. And while there may not be any visible manifestation of ill health, the experience of stress varies from person to person. It remains difficult to 'prove' to sceptical colleagues when one feels unable to turn up for work. While some nurses do express sympathy for their colleagues who feel they cannot take any more, they also feel 'if I can manage why can't she?'. Given the workload that nurses have to get through there is an implicit belief in everyone doing their fair share of the work. If they do not do their 'bit' then comments will be made. Hence the label 'bitchy'. 'You might get some bitchiness if you think someone is not pulling their weight and you're having sort of to carry them . . .' (Pupil). It is not easy to complain to a more senior nurse if someone is not working very hard but it is easy to mutter to the person you are working with. As senior nurses become more and more inaccessible, then grumbling to one's peers will increasingly become the only outlet for nurses. But there are dangers in conveying dissatisfactions or talking about problems to colleagues.

> I wasn't prepared to talk to anybody here [about a problem] in case it got back because I just thought if anything is said it will just make the situation totally worse. People never report it just the way you've said it, it's always altered and changed. (Staff Nurse)

Not only can accounts be distorted, the very fact that any complaint has been voiced may ensure that the label 'troublemaker' is assigned to you.

> . . . the people in the hierarchy do not like troublemakers, they like people to toe the line. (Staff Nurse)

> I'm not frightened of saying what I think, because I will say it if I'm not happy, I will say it and hope I will get respect from saying what I think. But I think if I said too much it wouldn't go down well and some people close ranks and you get labelled as a troublemaker. (Sister)

> Anyone extrovert is branded a troublemaker. Even though we are in 1987, if you speak out or have strong views you are asking for trouble. I'm the sort of person who tries to avoid arguments and confrontations at any cost. But even I have had my moments. (Enrolled Nurse)

Being labelled as a troublemaker can have many repercussions. It can affect promotion, being considered for further training, applications to move to another unit and many other career aspects.

> My Dad says why don't you turn round and tell her what you think of her. But you can't do that – at times you'd like to or give your point of view. But then if you want to leave, you want a reference and you're not going to get a good reference . . . And if you want to move onto another ward, they'll just turn round and be awkward. Or anything, holiday or whatever, they can just be awkward. Which is wrong really because they have just got us where they want us. (Enrolled Nurse)

> But I think people are so frightened of losing their jobs that nobody wants to be the first, and I'm as guilty as everybody else, to stand and actually say 'we're not having such-and-such . . .' (Sister)

A pupil nurse made quite clear the pressures learners were under to keep their comments which they put on the bottom of their final ward report to themselves:

> you can't really say all the things you want to say. Well I don't think you can because it follows you. Whatever anybody wrote

down – I know it's confidential – but people talk, don't they, like 'X is a troublemaker' because of what she had written when she had her report and they all went on and on about it.

The failure of learners to ask questions when being given their final ward report[6] is understandable. Not surprisingly, learners learn to keep quiet, and the giving of reports ends up as only one-way communication. The dislike of nurses who 'speak-out' is accompanied by the need to 'fit in': 'nursing is very much a profession where if your face fits you are all right' (Sister).

What sort of face does 'fit' depends in part on where you are and on the evaluation of colleagues that you have worked with. Your reputation is quickly built up and it precedes you when moving on to different allocations:

The theatre staff say 'we know all about you before you get here'. With it being so small, the ward staff know all about you before you arrive, so if you don't make a good impression on the ward, it could throw things a bit in theatre. (Alice)

There are a number of ways in which nurses are meant to behave.

When dealing with patients who were 'on the mend' I found that laughter was a great tonic and I endeavoured to lighten the atmosphere somewhat. In fact I got a good rollicking for singing whilst going about my duties as it wasn't professional! (Ex-Pupil-Nurse)

There's a lot of the old school with different expectations of how you should behave . . . whereas somebody my age loves the students to be, not cheeky exactly, but to have rapport with you . . . The older people can't cope with that because they are used to people doing as they were told. (Sister)

While changing jobs in order to gain a broad base in nursing, I came across some degree of suspicion as to why I did not 'settle to a job'. (Staff Nurse)

While senior nurses may have expectations of the way that nurses ought to behave, their own behaviour comes in for a substantial amount of criticism and is seen as lowering morale amongst nursing staff.

Some senior staff can go a bit too far. They are too critical, unapproachable and generally set a bad atmosphere on the ward. Unfortunately the patients suffer as well. (Staff Nurse)

An enrolled nurse's weekend was changed without consulting her when she was on holiday and when she queried it she was really snapped at and told 'Nurse so-and-so, if I say you have to work every weekend, then every weekend you will work'. Well that's disgraceful I think for somebody who has worked there that long and been a loyal member of staff. (Staff Nurse)

. . . we get no thanks for what we do at all and people need their morale boosting all the time, but they don't get it. (Staff Nurse)

The connection between the style of management of the most senior staff and those further down the hierarchy was made clearly by one sister:

If the leadership style is wrong it passes down the line and the nursing officer becomes apprehensive and defensive. This washes off on the sisters, etc. (Sister)

What appears to be an issue here is a lack of management skills amongst some of the more senior nurses. Some senior nurses exhibit a rather peremptory style of mangement which reinforces nurses' fear of 'speaking-out'. Similarly those senior nurses do not want to hear what their nurses have to say.

I just feel like they don't listen to you at all. You are not a person, you've not to complain. You will do as you are told, and you do because that's how you learn in school. You learn to take it, that's part of the training, you can't answer back, you've just got to take it. (Enrolled Nurse)

There are obvious difficulties for some nurses in expressing their opinions:

I would like to see regular meetings for all levels of staff and not very formal, because sometimes its very difficult to really be honest and very sure of your opinion. Small meetings, small informal meetings where you can really get down to proper people's feelings. (Staff Nurse)

A district nurse talked of one of the improvements she would like to see made:

To have people to turn to, to be able to talk to people and listen; people who are prepared to listen and don't just sort of listen to you for the sake of it and don't do anything about it. (District Nurse)

The need for some sort of counselling service, or someone to whom nurses could let off steam, was mentioned by a variety of nurses. Given the lack of care which they feel that senior nurses demonstrate, this finding is not surprising.

The support services given to nurses I think should be improved. I think there's very little for nurses. Like a nurse I have on here, he gets quite depressed, he's nowhere to go, there isn't a nursing support group or anything like that. (Acting Sister)

I think we could do with somebody . . . to air your views to – a great big punch bag in the corner so you can go in and tell them what you think. (Student)

The absence of counselling services which are completely in-dependent of the nursing hierarchy is to be bemoaned. There is an obvious, and often-expressed, demand for a counselling service from nurses. The need for counselling has been identified by many commentators.[7] Yet, few Health Authorities appear to offer in-dependent counselling services. The lack of such services implies a failure amongst senior nurse managers, who themselves are safely out of the clinical role, to recognize the stresses and strains involved in nursing today. A hierarchy unsympathetic to the needs of nurses may well end up facing a nursing workforce which is unsympathetic to the needs of management. The divisions within nursing between man-agers and nurses (exacerbated by the changes initiated as a result of the Griffiths recommendations[8]), become apparent. Thus Salvage can comment on the 'extraordinary lack of support and compassion for colleagues'.[9]

It must be emphasized that many of the more senior nurses do not lack management skills and try to ensure that a 'good atmosphere' prevails in their units.

The sisters are very nice, we are very fortunate on this ward. I think they are about the best that there is in the hospital – on this ward. We are very fortunate that they are both here. I think if it wasn't for the staff, how we buck each other up, we'd have all left a long time ago. (Staff Nurse)

On here it's really good . . . if you do anything wrong then you are told and you are not told in a nasty way, you are not taken into the office and the door shut . . . (Staff Nurse)

You get some wards that people sort of label: 'Oh, it's a bitchy ward' and things like that, but I've come across a lot more nicer ones than I have bad ones. (Student)

Of course, nurses differ in the expectations they have of one another and of one another's behaviour. Yet it appears that a common and influential factor in the demeanour of nurses is their training. The inability of many nurses to speak out and say what they think appears to have been learned during their nurse training.

> Nurses tend to have a subservient attitude to things such as low
> pay, long hours and arduous work – after all they are con-
> ditioned into it. (Enrolled Nurse)

> You're not trained to be assertive. I've seen senior nurses sitting
> back where they know a wrong decision is being made because
> they don't want to step out of line. (Staff Nurse)

It seems likely that if nurses felt more able to stand up and speak out
for themselves many of the problems regarding the 'bitchiness' of
nursing would be reduced. In an open atmosphere where criticism
can be constructively rather than destructively expressed, there is less
need to mutter and grumble behind others' backs.

> Nurses in general, older nurses especially, don't like change and
> tend to let things happen to us and I think we are our own worst
> enemy and we don't complain when we should. They will all
> chunter on behind their backs but they won't stand up and say
> anything. (Staff Nurse)

Much of this subservience can be linked to the relationship between
doctors and nurses. Nurses in the past have been seen and treated as
handmaidens: assisting the doctor and doing his bidding. The
expressing of opinions goes against the very nature of the relationship. It seems that a servile attitude is perpetuated by some of those
who train nurses. It is obvious that attitudes are changing, especially
amongst younger nurses. And it is the changing attitudes which
account for some of the reported frictions. A lack of self-esteem, and by
extension, a lack of esteem for colleagues, may exacerbate the
'atmosphere'. If nurses were given, and gave, greater respect the
atmosphere might improve. Ashley suggests that nurses' hostility to
one another is a reflection of misogynistic beliefs about women.[10]
Thus nurses, it is argued, have taken on board the attitudes of men
who are women-haters. The attitudes of influential colleagues, such
as doctors, can be misogynistic: attitudes which nurses may not have
questioned. Thus, for example, some nurses explain the 'bitchiness' in
nursing as the result of women working together.

'The atmosphere' within the ranks of nurses obviously is affected by
the style of management of nursing officers. (The role of nursing
officers will be looked at in greater detail in Chapter 8.) However,
working outside the clinical area, nursing officers lose the immediacy
of contact with the problems which daily face nurses. Yet, it is
expected that if a nurse has problems she or he will go to a senior
nurse: for many nurses that means going to a nursing officer. While
the majority of nurses felt they could go and talk to senior colleagues

about any work problems, there does seem to be a distinction between issues which are professional and those which are personal.[11]

> If it's to do with work, the nursing officer is very good, he'll deal with it there and then, no problem. To me if it is a personal problem from home then I'll deal with it at home. (Staff Nurse)

This distinction means that it is peers rather than senior nurses who are approached with personal problems. At the same time there appeared to be a lack of trust of some senior nurses.

> He's [nursing officer] a very nice man but when I've needed him he's not been there, he's not been very supportive. Especially with the trouble I had with the charge nurse but I didn't get any support then and I could have done with some really. (Sister)

Approaching a senior colleague may unduly formalize an issue:

> It's nice to have somewhere to go where you can discuss things, and know it's not like you are reporting somebody. But somewhere to discuss what to do about a situation. Because you do get things and there's loads of ways of handling them. And you just don't know which will be the best. (Acting Sister)

For nurses at sister level, choices as to who to go to with problems are very limited indeed. Sisters may have problems which are similar to those of junior nurses, yet they need to be managed in a different way.

> If I have a problem with my nursing officer, who do I go and talk to if it isn't one of my immediate colleagues – which then is very unprofessional. So we either come home and talk about it or talk amongst another group of sisters. But if we go to (the Director of Nursing Services) now that's too high, that isn't where you want to go, because you are not complaining at that level. You need something, an outlet but you don't want a formal outlet, you know, you don't want to start a chain of events. (Sister)

There is obviously a need for some other source of support for nurses at sister level. Suggestions were made by some sisters that informal sisters' meetings where more senior nurses were not present were needed. Thus, the support of colleagues who fully understand and appreciate the difficulties encountered by sisters could be obtained.

Although nursing officers may have a general influence on the atmosphere in a particular unit, it is a diffuse influence. A more direct and specific influence comes from the sister or charge nurse.[12] What makes a 'good sister'? The qualities which nursing officers feel makes a 'good' sister focus on many different skills but the qualities demanded of sisters revolve primarily around interpersonal skills. These skills are particularly important regarding the 'atmosphere' in which nurses work. I asked the nurses what made a good sister. (For the sake of simplicity, the word sister will be used to cover both sisters and charge nurses.) The most valued attribute was 'being approachable'

> The sisters are lovely, very approachable. They are willing to accept new ideas. They are quite young themselves but at the same time you respect them. You don't walk in fear of them, it's very nice. (Staff Nurse)

> Sister is excellent, very understanding. She is very approachable. She understands pupils and students and me as a first-year qualified nurse. (Enrolled Nurse)

> I like a sister that you don't feel frightened of but maybe they can still be a good sister when you are frightened of them anyway. I like one who keeps the rules, who sort of lays the ward out and says you do this, and you do that, an organized ward and she's very good with the patients, spends time with the patients and you can get on with her as a member of the staff; that I feel I can go to her and tell her if I had any problems. Like some sisters there's like a barrier between you. (Laura)

Also very highly valued was the willingness of sisters to roll up their sleeves and help out when their nurses were struggling to get all the work done.

> The sisters are very good to get on with here. They roll their sleeves up and get stuck in (Enrolled Nurse)

> I like sisters who won't ask you to do anything that they won't do themselves. I don't like somebody who sits behind a desk who just gives orders out and doesn't do anything themselves. (Barbara)

The need to establish a good relationship with the patients as well as with the staff was often mentioned.

> They need to be able to have a good relationship with the staff as well as with the patients. Not just the patients because it's the staff who keep it going. And if she doesn't get on with the staff . . .! (Wendy)

Sisters do not simply require interpersonal skills, they also need to have organizational skills. While, predictably, this aspect was most prominent in the views of nursing officers, all grades of nurses and learners mentioned the ability to organize.

They've got to be able to organize, to organize themselves and other people. Its surprising how many staff nurses look and think, well I do exactly what sister does, I can do it – but they can't. They've just got to have organizational ability, from the word go. (Nursing Officer)

Excellent organizational skills, the type of person who can tell someone what to do without beating around the bush, who can be quite firm. Assertiveness really. (Student)

To be understanding. I think you have got to be able to organize other people. You have to be able to cope with stress as well. And you have got to be able to cope with your nursing staff. I think you have got to be very level-headed. (Sheila)

Sisters clearly influence the atmosphere in a ward or unit. Nurses and learners are agreed on the need for a 'friendly' atmosphere. Nursing is stressful enough without the added difficulties of a tense atmosphere.

I hate it here, there's an atmosphere – everyone is unhappy . . . the sisters don't care, nobody bothers if you're not happy with something. A lot of it is to do with inexperienced staff – they don't know how to handle things and they're the sisters of the wards, the unit and they don't have a clue how to do things. This rubs off on the staff and nobody gives a damn now. (Enrolled Nurse)

At the same time, it is not good having a relaxed atmosphere if the work doesn't get done. Not only is there a need for organizing ability there is also a need to maintain the respect and a certain distance from the nursing staff. Respect was given for both 'putting a pinny on' and for running an efficient ward or unit.

I think you've definitely got to be approachable, but still remain, still have respect from the people who are under you or you wouldn't get anywhere. Yes, somebody who mucks in as well. I feel they do get more respect if they actually muck in and do the work. I don't think you get any respect for sitting in the office. (Ann)

I've worked for a very young Sister, who was absolutely excellent. She was a slave-driver but the ward was excellent. I didn't like her as a person but she ran an extraordinary ward. (Student)

It was clear that most nurses appreciated the difficulties under which sisters work. After all, many of the nurses themselves aspired to become sisters. There was obvious sympathy for the difficulties encountered by newly appointed and inexperienced sisters.

She's all right but she's just trying to find her feet. She had a lot of responsibilities put on her straight off and I think there was a lot of atmosphere, well bitchiness really, going on in the ward and she was just chucked in so she was really put in a difficult position. (Enrolled Nurse)

Nevertheless, particular deficiencies in the sisters' style of management were fairly frequently pointed out.

I found one of the charge nurses was not very helpful. Where I was working [in another hospital] you were given a lot more responsibility as a staff nurse. Here I find you have to go through channels for the slightest thing. (Staff Nurse)

I think all the sisters should go on managerial courses. A lot of them are good nurses and don't really know how to manage people. They are very offensive to student nurses and pupil nurses, you know if they are under stress . . . they don't think twice about sort of shouting right across [the unit] and making you feel about two inches high. And then everybody gets aggravated. (Staff Nurse)

Many of the perceived deficiencies in the activities of sisters related to managerial skills: devolution of responsibility, communication skills, motivating your staff, etc. The nursing officers in particular were well aware of the need for sisters to have a wide variety of management skills.

You've got to have a good leader. They've got to have leadership qualities. They have to have the ability to identify the needs on the wards. They have to have a lot of good qualities if they are going to be good sisters. Not only have they got to be good listeners, they've got to identify the needs, they've got to be sympathetic to the staff requests for off-duties . . . they have to be sympathetic towards the relatives of the patients . . . She has to be happy on that ward and if she's not happy with the standards of care the patients receive then she has to have the ability to realize it and what can be done about it. She has to be able to cope with emergencies, the consultants and every department in the hospital . . . It really is a very demanding position.

I think one thing they've got to have is a sense of humour because if they don't they are really going to go down, it's a battle otherwise – you are just battling with yourself and everybody . . . I think they've got to have had good experience in their specialty because they are asked so much about it and they need to know. They need to be good at communication because they do communicate at all levels. And they've got to be able to take stress.

The interpersonal skills which are so important a part of the sister's work are essentially management skills. A lack of training opportunities for all nurses was mentioned in Chapter 6. The lack of management training is important not only from the perspective of individual nurses who wish to gain promotion but also in the day-to-day working relationships in the wards and elsewhere. All nurses lose out by the failure to develop nurses in managerial roles. It is a failure which is most evident in the morale and the grumbling atmosphere to be found within nursing. 'Bitchiness' is a reflection of operating difficulties such as too tight staffing levels and inadequate management skill development amongst sisters. Nursing officers also have a role to play in the atmosphere of a unit. However, most responsibility for the atmosphere in a ward must lie with the sister.

A lot of it [the atmosphere] comes from the top. It comes from the sister and works down. That's what I found both as a student and as a nurse manager. It depends how the sister sees nursing; how she runs the wards; how she sees the staff; how she keeps them. I think she's the king-pin really. No matter what you are looking at really, she is the key person. (Nursing Officer)

The sister is absolutely all important on a ward. (Student)

I think it does stem from the sister to start with. If the sister is disorganized, doesn't know what she is doing or isn't a very good planner, etc. then the nurses just don't feel they are fulfilling their role properly, not quite sure of when the job begins and ends I think. (Nursing Officer)

No matter how important sisters are for the morale and atmosphere amongst nurses there are definite limits to their responsibility. Sisters do not choose to work with tight staffing levels, with increasing workloads, with nurses who are frustrated through lack of promotion, training prospects, etc. They have to bear the brunt of the 'cost-efficiencies' which are being attempted by the government in the NHS at the moment. The widespread existence of bitchiness and low morale is an indication of sisters' inability to contain the effects of the 'efficiencies' being imposed on them. Sisters have an unenviable job. At least their colleagues are generally aware of this.

Notes

1 DHSS (1972), p. 34.
2 Annandale-Steiner (1979), p. 36, Salvage (1985), p. 71.

3 Peach L. (1986) 'Manpower and personnel policies: the national perspective', *Hospital and Health Services Review*, September, 82:5, p. 204.
4 Submission by ACAS *in* Merrison (1979), p. 463.
5 Tuckett (ed.) (1976), p. 239.
6 See also Mathieson, A. (1984) 'Wasted opportunities', *Nursing Mirror*, 8 February, p. 23.
7 Birch (1975), p. 80, DHSS (1972), pp. 176–8, Royal College of Nursing (1978b) *Counselling*, London, RCN; Salvage (1985), p. 166.
8 Griffiths, E.R. (1983) *NHS Management Enquiry*, London, DHSS.
9 Salvage (1985), p. 14.
10 Ashley, J.A. (1980) 'Power in structured misogyny' *Advances in Nursing Science*, 2:3, p. 20.
11 RCN (1978b), p. 53.
12 Research on hospital sisters is reported by Redfern (1980) and Redfern, S.J. and Spurgeon, P. (1980) 'Job satisfaction and withdrawal of hospital sisters in the UK' *in* Duncan, K.D., Gruneberg, M.M. and Wallis, D. *Changes in Working Life*, London, Wiley.

8

Who Looks After the Nurses?

'They call nursing the caring profession but, you know, who does care for the carers?' (Student).

There is little doubt that nursing is a demanding occupation which becomes a way of life rather than just a job. Work spills over into leisure, the professional merges with the personal life of nurses. Yet nurses' need for an 'independent ear' at work is not met. The unsympathetic hierarchy within nursing together with a perceived lack of management skills in nurse managers leaves nurses with no protectors. Nurses feel their nurse managers, their administrators, and the government have failed them. The special relationships previously enjoyed within nursing have been eroded. The role played by trade unions and professional associations leaves something to be desired. Nurses feel isolated as they come to be treated increasingly as an industrial workforce. The failure of the trade unions to meet the needs of nurses is due partly to the attitude of nurses themselves to collective, political action. It is also likely to reflect a past disinterest in women and part-time workers in the wider trade union movement.

Nursing is not an easy job. It is both stressful and tiring. The morale of the nursing workforce is not high. There is a 'grumbling atmosphere' and complaints of bitchiness. What effect does this have on nurses?

Three-quarters of the nurses felt their social life was affected by nursing. Most often mentioned were the shifts, the hours and the associated tiredness.

My hobbies are fell-walking, mountaineering, orienteering and things like that, something we do very much at the weekend as a family . . . I didn't realize that I would miss it quite as much, that

> I would miss doing things with them quite so much, because we work two out of three weekends. (Sister)

> Apart from being on nights, you find you are too tired to go out sometimes; too tired to be bothered talking to people, especially after a 10-day stretch. If you've been working 10 days in a row and you get to day 7 and that's it, you can't be bothered talking to people, you are very bad tempered, unbearable to live with basically . . . you get very edgy. (Student)

Working weekends, working nights, having rotas changed at the last moment all affect the activities of many nurses. It is difficult to make plans and to keep 'dates'. It is also a problem if your friends or partner have 9–5 jobs.

> If you are only finishing working at 9 o'clock and your husband says 'shall we go out for a drink?' You think I'd rather put my feet up for an hour, I'd rather go to bed, I'm at work in the morning you know . . . And it's very hard sometimes to say 'can I not just stop in with a cup of cocoa?' because he's finished work at 5 o'clock and he's had 4 hours to put his feet up or do what he wanted to do. (Staff Nurse)

The way in which nurses spend their leisure time can be affected as well. With shift patterns that vary from week to week it is difficult, if not impossible, to attend classes on a weekly basis:

> . . . if my husband could get transferred to days I was going to start going to nightschool with him . . . and do some more O levels or an A level. But then I'd have to start arranging my off-duty around that. You see you are very restricted in what you can do, you've got to arrange your social life around your hours. Or muck up the off-duty for everybody else. But you can't close a hospital down at 5 o'clock. (Staff Nurse)

The difficulties of attending nightschool were mentioned by many nurses. It is a particular problem for enrolled nurses who wish to obtain the necessary extra O and A levels to become registered nurses. There are, of course, problems and constraints for anyone who works shifts. But nursing causes special problems because the shifts do not necessarily follow a consistent pattern. In the psychiatric hospital the (12-hour) shifts did follow a set pattern and nurses found it so much easier to plan their social lives. Indeed, the shifts hardly seemed to affect them at all. It is not clear why general nursing with its shorter shifts cannot be similarly arranged. For the moment, 'doing the rota' is one of the most disliked tasks which sisters have to do. It is time-consuming and it is difficult fitting in individuals' requests for specific days off.

Only a handful of nurses felt that their social life actually benefited from working the odd shifts.

> I enjoy working weekends, having time off during the week. We do work late shifts so if you work till 5 one day and you're not on until dinner the next day it's better than 9–5 jobs because you can go out, you've got a lie-in the next day. I prefer working the shifts . . . (Staff Nurse)

Also, some nurses said their leisure activities were positively enhanced by working shifts. They were off work when others were not. As a result the shops and the leisure facilities were quiet when they were off duty. Some favour this while others yearn for 'normality'.

> If I wasn't a nurse I'd be perhaps doing a 9–5 job so I would just have evenings and weekends off, whereas at the moment I can have days off during the week, 4 days together. You know I quite like the hours and the way I work – it means I can play golf if I want to, or go out in the garden, if the weather is nice . . . (Sister)

While there may be problems in fitting in with those who work 'normal' hours, the shifts can have advantages for those with families.

> I think the children see more of me than they ever would do if I was in a 9–5 job when they'd only ever see me at weekends. I'm home quite a lot during the day. (Male Staff Nurse)

Working as a nurse involves a great deal more than just working odd hours. As was shown in Chapter 5 the vast majority of nurses find it a stressful job. How do nurses deal with that stress? Is there someone they can go and talk to?

Partners, friends and colleagues

In spite of the comments which had been made earlier about the bitchy atmosphere in nursing over a quarter said they could deal with their stress by talking to colleagues.

> Me? I swear. And I have good colleagues that I talk to. We talk to each other, which is very good as we all understand each other. And if we are fed up or tired or whatever we talk it out and it usually comes out OK. (Charge Nurse)

> Mainly I think with talking to colleagues that understand. Because there's no point in going home and saying: 'Oh I've had

an awful day' to friends because they just say: 'Well, so have I, so what?' And I think it's only people that know what the pressures are like that can sympathize. Unless you've been in that situation and you know what somebody is talking about, it doesn't mean anything. And you think well she understands because she's been through it herself, or he has. (Sister)

Talking to colleagues and getting rid of stress means that nurses are more likely to be able to leave their work at work. For some, work finishes when they walk out the door. They have learned to switch themselves off:

I never used to be able to do. I used to go home and think I've not done this and I've not done that but not now. I just switch off when I walk out. (Enrolled Nurse)

For others it is impossible to leave their work. They take it home with them. Once home, there are a number of ways in which nurses do manage to let off steam. Most often it is partners or flatmates who have to listen as nurses wind down from their working day.

I go home and I have a good moan to my husband. He will listen, he's great really, you know. He discusses it with me and I calm down. (Enrolled Nurse)

At home, because my husband is a nurse anyway and he knows exactly what it's like anyway. It must be difficult explaining to someone who is not a nurse the sort of things you may have seen that day. (Sister)

It is not always easy for partners and friends to listen and undoubtedly some strain is carried over into the relationship.

I talk it through with my friend who I live with and that helps. Before that I used to go home and it caused stress at home because I was taking it out on my Mum and Dad because I wasn't prepared to talk to anybody here in case it got back. (Staff Nurse)

Various activities help nurses relieve their tensions and the problems from work: rugby, running, riding, walking the dog, a visit to the pub. Friends are often called in to help. The most helpful friends are those who are nurses.

Two of my closest friends are nurses and we go out and we perhaps talk about things that have happened at work and if you are feeling a failure you often find that they have had a similar experience and you don't feel as bad. (Staff Nurse)

Quite a few nurses said they had no outlet for their stress. For one or another reason they bottle up their feelings or they can't get rid of them.

> Well I don't have any outlet really because I'm a single parent, on my own with a small child. (Health Visitor)

> I can't switch off. If I've worked a late duty and with being busy I don't particularly sleep that night because there are still things racing around. I just can't do it, I just can't switch off and my husband says you should come out of work and you should forget about it but I can't do that. (Sister)

> You do go to bed sometimes and you can still hear babies crying and if you've had a sad occasion – a death or something like that, it does tend to stay with you for a while, but you've just got to . . . You get a run of really poorly children sometimes and it can be really upsetting, stressful. (Staff Nurse)

The need to talk to someone who understands and appreciates the particular demands of nursing was apparent from many of the nurses' comments on this topic. Sympathetic noises from a friend or partner who doesn't really understand the particular demands of nursing seem to be a poor substitute for talking to another nurse. Quite a number bemoaned that fact that there was nowhere or no one at work to whom they felt they could go and talk.

> It would not be a bad idea if there was somebody who could listen to your problems and advise you on them. Somebody who wasn't involved on the unit. It would be a nice change to be able to go to somebody. You tend to go to a close friend and have a good moan. If you feel what you say could get back, you end up saying nothing. (Enrolled Nurse)

> [Nurses] are very frightened to speak out. Well, I'm frightened. I don't always say what I think. I just sort of take it all home and moan about it to everybody else. (Student)

> I think there should be like a helpline or something that you could phone up and without mentioning names, or patients' names, or anything like that, just say: 'Oh, and this bloke arrested today and it was really awful.' Just somebody who would sit on the other end of the phone and say: 'Oh that's terrible, oh yes, I know how you feel' and if it was nurses on the other end of the phone . . . (Staff Nurse)

The need for some sort of support service of helpline was frequently expressed. Not only do nurses have problems dealing with the particular demands of the job, but like anyone else, they have personal problems. Just as it is sometimes difficult to leave work problems at work, so it may be difficult to leave personal problems at home. If hospitals are large and impersonal, it is not easy for personal relationships to be built up. Sitting alone over dinner and recognizing few faces in the canteen or in the corridors can make problems at home or at work seem much larger. And nurses who are worried or concerned about something are less likely to do their job well. Trying to care for or comfort a patient is particularly stressful when you are needing some care and comfort yourself. The provision of some sort of confidential counselling service for nurses would undoubtedly be of great benefit. In a large hospital with hundreds of nurses, the cost benefits of such a scheme would probably mean that it paid for itself. From many different directions the need for a comprehensive counselling service emerged. It remains, 17 years after Briggs, a 'top priority'.[1]

One of the major requirements in setting up a counselling service is that the service needs to be completely independent of the nursing hierarchy. Too often counselling implies, because it has previously taken place within the hierarchical nursing structure, a 'dressing-down'.[2] Although the support of supervisors has been found elsewhere to reduce 'burn-out'[3] as well as amongst nurse learners,[4] in nursing there are barriers to using senior colleagues for support. Real, or imagined, lack of respect for confidences amongst senior colleagues ensures that approaches are not made without great thought.[5] From aspects ranging from learners' ward reports to complaints regarding unprofessional behaviour, it is evident that, for some nurses at least, the nursing hierarchy is not trusted.

Nursing officers

The role of nursing officer is not an enviable one. Drawn from the ranks of nurses, the use of the term 'nursing' in the job title is a misnomer. Nursing officers have little or no clinical involvement. First and foremost they are managers and administrators.[6] Nurses who wish to become managers must leave the clinical area. Such a move may present problems for someone who entered nursing in order to nurse. Many of the nursing officers spoke of missing patient contact (but not all of whom would, however, consider returning to clinical nursing!). The distancing of nursing officers from clinical involvement is often not liked by other nurses.

A significant number of nurses feel their superiors to be uncaring about the welfare of their nurses. One-third of the nurses were critical of their nursing officer. The criticisms focused on three main areas: not being assertive enough, not backing-up the nursing staff, and a general lack of interest or care in the nursing staff.

They are either not assertive enough or they are power-mad. Mrs X is a lovely person but she cannot come out and say what she means because she wants to be loved by everyone. (Staff Nurse)

She's not the sort of person I feel that you could go to with a problem because she just has no consideration for staff at all, as long as her numbers are right that's all she's worried about. (Enrolled Nurse)

I personally would like to have seen her [nursing officer] out in the community more – she is based in the hospital and she rarely comes out into the community . . . Occasionally you do feel very much on your own, you get a bad social problem, something like that and sometimes you feel you would just like somebody else to come and give their views on it. She tends to throw it very much back at us, you know, she will say: 'Well, I know you can cope with it.' Which is nice, but . . . (Sister)

No, she is not approachable. She has a very domineering attitude. She tends to make a decision and doesn't like it being questioned. She will do things for the smooth running of the department, without a lot of consideration for the nursing staff. (Sister)

As with sisters, the nursing officer who got 'stuck in' and helped on the ward or with the work was much appreciated. But it was this aspect which, in particular, pointed to the inherent difficulties in the role of nursing officers. Promotion at sister level means moving into management and moving out of clinical work. Nursing officers may quickly lose touch with clinical developments or practices. The clinical skills of an experienced sister or health visitor may be greater than those of the nursing officer.[7] At the same time it is not always clear that nursing officers have been adequately prepared for their job. Some of the nursing officers I talked to reported that they felt they had been 'thrown in at the deep end'. The issues involved were noted by one sister:

I feel many of the problems in nursing have been caused by the career pattern that has been offered for many years. Promotion only comes from entering nurse administration. Many good ward sisters were coerced into becoming nursing officers. They were not always good nursing officers because their job satisfaction was lost and the established nursing administration had not

ensured that correct career counselling and management training were given.

The type of management training offered to nursing officers tends to
be short modules of, at most, a few weeks' duration. While there
appeared to be general agreement that there were enough training
opportunities for short courses, the scarcity of substantial management courses was mentioned.

> I don't think we have enough management training but I feel it
> must be a nurse who does the job because she needs to know the
> patients, the care and to know how the staff functions. But I
> really do feel that probably there should be a year or 2 years out of
> nursing to go and do a proper management degree course. I
> really feel you need that.

There are complaints about training at sister level and a general
dissatisfaction with opportunities for nurses to train further. At the
same time, while nursing officers are offered a range of courses it is not
clear they receive an appropriate level of management training. As
with the more junior grades of nurses, there is no financial incentive
for nursing officers to go for further training. Again this is a somewhat
short-sighted policy which does not ensure that the talents and skills
of senior members of the workforce are fully developed. As with the
general lack of training opportunities which other nurses felt, the
gender of the workforce may have had a role to play in determining
the level of training even at manager level. Of course, throughout
Britain there is a lamentable lack of interest in management training.[8]

Despite the criticisms, many nursing officers were seen positively by
the nursing workforce. And, most nursing officers were happy with
their job. They felt that they had been adequately prepared for their
job and it was also a promotion that they had actively pursued.
Similarly, some nursing officers had become used to the greatly
reduced contact with patients that came with their job.

> At first it was awful, if I think about it, the first few months, I kept
> thinking I should go back just because of that [patient contact]
> but now, no, you get used to it. The job has changed so much and
> it's more challenging and I enjoy it. So I've changed myself I
> suppose and you realize that you have a different role altogether.

For some nursing officers, the lack of patient contact was regretted.

> If I had my time over again I would not do this. I would have
> stayed a sister. But I don't know if I could have coped with the
> physical work . . . But I really feel I've got away from what I
> wanted to do.

Nursing officers have to face two ways at once. They have to address themselves to problems of management and administration but they also have to concern themselves with clinical matters. There is a tension in their work which is not always easily resolved. It is a tension which is reflected in the complaints of nurses about nursing officers. Nurses think that nursing officers should somehow be 'on their side'. The Director of Nursing Services, on the other hand, has appointed nursing officers as managers and administrators. In trying to meet the demands of both, nursing officers may end up doing neither well. A nursing officer who gives a great deal of attention to the nursing workforce may find that she is being negatively judged regarding her administrative and managerial work. As a result, the nursing officer is unlikely to have much 'clout' when putting forward demands on behalf of the nursing workforce. Similarly, a nursing officer who is 'all for management' fails in the eyes of the nurses. Lacking credibility, any changes which such a nursing officer tries to make at ward or unit level is more likely to be resisted by the nursing workforce. It is not surprising that some nursing officers fall between the two stools. The repercussions of this are to be found in the unwillingness of some nurses to go to their nursing officer with their problems.

Another part of the difficulty regarding nursing officers, as mentioned in Chapter 7 is the distinction that is made between professional and personal problems.[9] Personal problems, it appears, are not the concern of nursing officers. For some nurses, this is an acceptable stance; others seem to feel somewhat let down:

> I can go to her [the nursing officer] professionally about anything, but personally I would never go to her because she's not really interested in that side of her nursing staff, I feel. (Sister)

Three factors appear to be involved in this somewhat artificial distinction between personal and professional. Firstly, there is a lack of empathy with nurses who do have problems. It is not simply an uncaring attitude, it also reflects the sentiment that 'good nurses' don't complain, they suffer in silence.[10] It is 'unprofessional' to complain. A second factor is a lack of interpersonal and communication skills amongst senior nurses. In essence this results from a lack of training in management skills. In turn the sorely felt needs of the workforce can be ignored or dismissed. A third factor, is the importance of the distinctions in rank amongst nurses. This may seem strange given that many of the more experienced nurses will 'act-up' for their immediate superior. But obedience, deference and a respect for authority are built into nurse training. And they are habits which die hard amongst the ranks of qualified nurses. The autocratic hierarchy is 'strong and pervasive'.[11] The somewhat military style of many aspects of nursing are overlaid with unwritten class distinctions which have been retained from earlier days. The divisive elements within nursing[12] ensure that many nurses fail to find a sympathetic ear.

Although immediate nursing colleagues may act as a support for nurses (see Chapter 7), successful attempts to achieve support from the nursing hierarchy appear to be few and far between. There appears to be a lack of care for the nurses working at 'the sharp end'. To some extent this reflects the difficulties inherent in the position of senior nurses. The inability for senior nurses to be involved in clinical work has been bemoaned by members of the medical profession.[13] It ought also to be bemoaned by those who would wish nurses to have rather more support from their seniors.

The present cost-efficiency savings which are being made in the Health Service also contribute to the problems facing nursing officers. They have to implement changes which may involve increasing the workload, reducing any 'slack' in the staffing levels, and generally seeking economies on the nursing side. It appears that, increasingly, nursing officers are having to distance themselves from the perspective of nurses and move ever closer to a management viewpoint. Such a movement may not be to the long-term advantage of nursing officers.

In the health authority the numbers of nursing officers had recently been much reduced. In future they are to be called Nurse Managers. Their title will be reflected in their job content. Increasing their workload, nurse managers will have less and less 'slack' in their own jobs to 'walk the wards' or make visits to health centres, etc. They have been further withdrawn from the everyday concerns of nurses. And it is likely that they will increasingly present a management rather than a nursing orientation towards nurses.

It was obvious that nursing officers were often used as scapegoats for all the problems currently being felt in the health authority. Nursing officers, being the first rank beyond clinical nursing bore the brunt of dissatisfactions. With the move towards nurse *managers*, the amount of 'stick' that these ex-nurses will have to take will increase.

With the introduction of general managers and the divisions between nurse managers and clinical nurses, nurses have increasingly become a workforce to be 'managed'. It appears that nurses, along with other health-care workers are to be treated as an industrial workforce. However, by treating the workforce as an industrial one they overlook the substantial goodwill that has existed amongst health-care workers towards the NHS. It has been pointed out that the feeling of 'family' which existed in the Health Service is being eroded.[14] What the workforce has, in the past, given freely and out of commitment to the NHS may be withheld when cheese-paring cuts are being experienced in every specialty. A management which deals only in monetary terms may well end up with a workforce that only works for monetary rewards – not a happy prospect for the workforce or their clients.

Nurses feel that no one is looking after their interests – or the interests of the patients. The special relationships which have existed throughout all the levels in the nursing hierarchy in the past are being damaged. The amount of distrust between manager and managed is likely to increase. At the same time it would be surprising if the amount of active discontent, such as higher absence, less willingness to work beyond 'finishing time' etc. did not increase. Many of those working in the NHS feel themselves to have a special vocation for their work. If they are treated as though they were the same as any other workforce: if their commitment was ignored or denied; then the goodwill on which the NHS depends would diminish. This, of course, may not be unpalatable to those who wish to see an extension of the private health-care sector.

Managers and administrators

Beyond nurses in the Health Service, are the managers and administrators. They are not viewed positively by the nurses. The sympathies of managers are not thought to be with the nursing workforce. There is a substantial degree of antagonism to the management. The introduction of general mangers comes in for a great deal of criticism as does the introduction of managers who are not nurses.

I think management do what they want to do regardless of who it upsets and who it hurts and whatever it means. I think management decide and that's it, tough if you don't like it. (Sister)

It bugs me that nursing seems to be so top heavy. When you go into the dining room all you seem to see are administrators and office workers – you hardly see any nurses there. I think many people feel that money is being taken away from the nursing side and going into administration. (Staff Nurse)

I don't approve of all these people coming in to the top posts who know absolutely nothing about hospitals. That does annoy me a lot. (Sister)

You're just a number, they couldn't care less. (Enrolled Nurse)

A good number of nurses said they knew so little about the management and administration that they could make no comment. From the comments that were received few were made from first-hand contact.

There is little doubt that local management/administration were being blamed for the many changes taking place in the Health Authority. While, nursing officers have, and for some considerable time, acted as scapegoats for problems experienced in the clinical areas, they are being increasingly joined by 'the management' at district headquarters. There is no doubt that the management was responsible for initiating a number of economies which were affecting the nurses directly. But it was the management which was getting the blame for the cash limits which had been imposed by the government on the Health Authority. In a similar fashion, changes which had been initiated at Director of Nursing Services level were blamed on the management and administration at district headquarters. It seems that by focusing on local management, attention is, to some extent, diverted away from government policies regarding the Health Service. Attention is also diverted away from the role played by senior nurses in participating in implementing these 'efficiency' measures.

It was evident that few nurses felt that management was 'on their side'. Of course, to the extent that managers have not previously worked in the Health Service, there is criticism that 'How can they know what patients need?' In the past, nurses seem to have felt they had allies in management. With the introduction of 'general' managers, the movement away from managers with direct patient involvement or experience accelerated. There is a tension, in other words, between managerial values and the caring values of nurses orientated to the needs of patients.[15] A few nurses feel unable to talk about their problems to colleagues, and many feel that senior nurses do not have the interests of nurses at heart. Similarly, nurses feel that management are not interested in their welfare. Given that many nurses feel isolated and lacking in support at work, is there anywhere else they can go for assistance?

Professional associations and trade unions:

The vast majority of nurses belong to a professional organization or to a trade union.[16] The most popular body amongst nurses is the Royal College of Nursing (RCN). Over half of the nurses belonged to the RCN. (Historically, trade unions were introduced into nursing through the assimilation of male asylum attendants into the occupation. Until 1960, men were excluded from membership of the RCN.)[17] COHSE, the Confederation of Health Service Employees accounted for less than one-fifth of the nurses. Only a very small proportion were members of The Royal College of Midwives (RCM) and the National Union of Public Employees (NUPE). The Health Visitors Association (HVA) was also occasionally mentioned.

Despite the high level of professional body or trade union membership, nurses rarely regarded their 'union' representative as someone they could simply go and talk to. When contact with the union representative was sought it was normally as the result of a specific event. The large majority of nurses (over two-thirds) felt that their union *was* looking after their interests. Around a quarter of nurses viewed their union negatively. The most common complaint was that the union was not forceful enough.

> The RCN is an utter waste of time, money and effort – a lame bulldog with no teeth. (Student)

> Well I think it's [the RCM] very good for what it is – it's informative for midwives. I don't know that it does a lot for improving midwives' pay . . . (Staff Nurse)

The charge of being out of touch with members' needs was levelled by a small number of nurses. While some attention was paid to the union's national performance, the most important factor in satisfaction with the union appeared to be the calibre of the representative. One COHSE representative received fulsome praise from many colleagues.

> COHSE is very good. They are more militant than the RCN. The RCN sit back and say 'well it is wrong' but don't do anything about it. But COHSE will fight for you – their union rep is marvellous. (Staff Nurse)

> Well the [COHSE] union rep was working on the next ward and he'd often come over but I've never really used the union, but he kept us up to date. He was very good. (Enrolled Nurse)

Despite the high level of union membership, the union representative was very seldom the person that nurses 'let off steam to'. Indeed, only one nurse, who was in NUPE, mentioned it: 'the sisters will listen but that is as far as it goes. I think your union representative is probably the one who listens most' (Staff Nurse). Interest in unions is very desultory amongst nurses. Most just seem to pay their subscriptions and leave the union to it. Students and pupils are advised to join a

union 'for their own protection' in the event of a dispute or unfair
dismissal etc. But according to the learners, the unions showed little
interest in recruiting them.

> I joined the RCN. I don't really hear that much from it. I think all
> of us joined, of those that did join the union . . . the RCN had the
> membership forms and nobody else came to see us. (Theresa)

> You pay your money and you get a slip quarterly and that's
> about it. (Wendy)

It is not surprising that there is such a low level of interest in union
activities if little enthusiasm is to be found amongst the representatives and other members. Given the many problems and areas of
discontent that nurses have mentioned, there is potentially a large
and influential role for unions to play. Union representatives are
uniquely placed to listen to and voice the concerns and difficulties
facing nurses. At the moment in this Health Authority they seldom
appear to be playing other than a passive role.

Having asked how nurses might get a better deal for themselves, a
non-unionized staff nurse replied:

> I've no idea really, they need somebody to adopt them and sort of
> fight for their cause. But how they would go about it themselves I
> don't know – I think they are very limited in what they can do
> themselves. (Staff Nurse)

Perhaps it is time that the various nursing associations and unions
started doing more for the nurses at local level than merely taking
their money. Yet, it has been noted elsewhere that senior staff may
make it clear that trade union activities amongst nurses are not
welcome.[18] There are other barriers to trade unions winning the
hearts of nurses. Very seldom were any political arguments presented
in conversation by the nurses I spoke to. Nurses do not appear to be a
'political' group of people. Indeed, it seems that many nurses actively
shun any contact with political views. Partly this may be due, as
Salvage suggests that the image of nurses as 'angels' almost precludes
them taking 'their destiny into their own hands'.[19] The 'good nurse' is
one who doesn't complain. By extension, the good nurse is one who
doesn't rock the boat, especially through holding strong political
views. There are other difficulties for trade unions in seeking to act
effectively on behalf of nurses. Firstly, all grades of nurses, including
learners, are to be found, for example, in the RCN. This results in
complaints from those in the ranks that the RCN is 'more for the
senior nurses'. Yet a complementary complaint can be heard from
nursing officers:

I had a grievance taken out against me [unsuccessfully] and when I had to go to the grievance hearing I found that the person was also in the RCN and I must admit I sat there thinking, well, 'they should be representing me as well instead of going against me', because I am also in the same union, and there was my union, against me . . . (Nursing Officer)

The presence of senior nurses at meetings may 'blunt the edge of legitimate criticism by junior staff . . .'.[20] Again, the notion of 'professionalism' acts against a commitment to trade unions. 'The RCN and its ilk are labelled as professional, patient-orientated, caring and good, while the TUC unions are supposed to be unprofessional, worker-orientated, selfish and bad.'[21] The idea of professionalism also acts to prevent alliances with non-nursing health service workers.[22] In this view, the interests of the profession are seen as somehow being different to those of other NHS employees.

Of course, trade unions have not, until recently, accommodated themselves to the fact that most of their members or potential members, are women.[23] Similarly, a system of workplace representatives has only recently been developed by the RCN (as a result of the competition from growing membership in trade unions)[24] through which support can potentially be given to individual nurses.

The government

Given that the professional associations and trade unions do not, as yet, play a particularly supportive role for individual nurses, is there anyone else looking after the interests of nurses? Are nurses' employers at national level, the government, looking after their interests? In response to my question, it appears that the nurses do not seem to think the government is looking after their interests.

The government doesn't seem to be caring for the nurses. (Enrolled Nurse)

We are supposed to be a professional group but we do not get treated like any other professionals. It is very degrading and upsetting. I know my future in nursing is very bleak. If the NHS continue to treat us the way they do, I will not continue working for them. (Pupil)

In fact, government policies are blamed for most of the problems encountered by nurses in their day-to-day work. In particular the staffing levels and the lack of funds to improve those levels are mentioned.

> It's part of the overall philosophy, you know, . . . nurses are the biggest single section, so we are the prime targets for cuts. (Charge Nurse)

> I think the time is coming when the public will have to be made aware that the cutbacks in nursing services are affecting their lives. I don't know where the figures come from that the government quote – I know they keep saying that they've put X number of more nurses into the system, but I don't know where they are . . . the system is continuing at a satisfactory level but simply because the nurses are working to their absolute maximum capacity. (Sister)

The standards of care, the ward closures, the lack of equipment are also blamed on the government and its financial restrictions on the NHS.

> Governmental restraint on finances cause us to close wards and decline to take on certain treatments. (Enrolled Nurse)

> The policies of the present government are having a catastrophic effect on the NHS, particularly I feel for the provisions for care for the mentally ill, and especially the chronic mentally ill . . . (Staff Nurse)

> The NHS is used as a political tool by certain political parties. I feel that a deterioration in the service we can offer to the public has taken place and continues unabated. I don't feel we will ever regain the lost ground in health care and facilities. (Staff Nurse)

> The letters come round every week saying this has got to happen and that's got to cut down. Obviously she [the Director of Nursing Services] gets it from somebody else. I mean she can't help it – it all comes from Margaret Thatcher, doesn't it? (Enrolled Nurse)

There is no doubt that many nurses feel the government is not on their side and is not looking after their interests. Many comments have been made regarding the difficulties of 'speaking-out' in nursing, talking to colleagues and senior nurses, and an uncaring management. It should, therefore, come as no surprise that many nurses feel they are very much 'on their own'. It is another factor which contributes to the low morale and grumbling atmosphere within the ranks of nursing. So, who does care for the nurses?

> Nobody. I don't think anybody really cares for us. Hospital management don't seem to care. And if they do they are probably that limited in what they can do . . . (Enrolled Nurse)

No one apart from our relatives. Our poor relatives get it every night when we go home. 'I'm sick of being taken for a mug. I'm sick of being put on all the time. Why don't they give us more staff, why can't they give us any more money? – They must be sick of hearing us. (Staff Nurse)

I don't think anybody does. We've got to muddle through on our own. (Staff Nurse)

In England, people who care about other people are definitely in the minority . . . England, at the moment is not a caring society. (Staff Nurse)

Strike?

Nurses do need champions because many feel their own hands are tied. The majority of nurses say they will not go on strike.

I don't think anybody really would fight for us and we can't do it ourselves because it would mean striking and that is one thing we can't do. (Enrolled Nurse)

These nurses say they do not want to go on strike because it would harm their patients. And part of the attraction of the Royal College of Nursing as a professional body for many nurses is its no-strike policy. But at the same time nurses were aware of the lack of tactical strength this involved.

I think a lot of the nurses wouldn't [strike]. Because it would be on their conscience and I think the government knows this . . . I think they know they've got us over a barrel. (Enrolled Nurse)

The fear of speaking out is important here. Many nurses are frightened of the repercussions (from within the ranks of nursing) if they stand up and say their piece. The strength of the no-strike ethos ensures that the more timid spirits stay in their place.

That's what's wrong with nurses, for too long they have been the underdogs. And I don't know if it's being frightened of victimiz-ation, I really don't know why nowadays they won't stand up and speak for themselves. I mean a few will but you don't need a few, you need everybody. You need a concerted voice. I don't know how you get nurses to do that. (Sister)

A small minority of nurses are prepared to go on strike and they have usually voted wth their feet and left the RCN to join a more militant union. 'I would go on strike. I think that's the only way at this moment in time that we're actually going to get anywhere' (Staff Nurse). Even some RCN members said they might now consider taking strike action.

> A year ago I would have said no, but I'd consider it now. Because we are falling behind, we are not able to maintain the standards. OK, pay is part of it but it's standards as well. I don't know, unless something is done to attract more people to the profession soon then it will be in a terrible state. (Charge Nurse)

However, most nurses still feel unable to strike and to leave their patients. A ballot of RCN members in March 1988[25] which showed a substantial majority against strike action which could put patients at risk. Additional pressure not to strike is exerted by the threatened exclusion from the recommendations of the Pay Review Body of any groups taking industrial action. They would consider other tactics: not carrying out any non-nursing duties, off-duty picketing, demonstrations, etc. But without the threat of striking, nurses are fairly powerless to effect any changes in their or the NHS's conditions. Perhaps the only solution is for other workers to stand up and shout on behalf of nurses: 'No, I would never go on strike . . . I think other people should go on strike for us, like porters and cleaners' (Patricia). Support for the nurses has been forthcoming from some groups of non-NHS workers, such as bus crews, dockers, and miners. Perhaps the general public also should start defending their National Health Service and the nurses who care for them. It is strange that there is an expectation that it is the providers rather than the receivers of health care who should defend the NHS.

Notes

1 DHSS (1972), p. 176.
2 RCN (1978b), p. 17.
3 Maslach, C. (1976) 'Burned-out', *Human Behaviour*, September, 5, p. 20.
4 Firth *et al.* (1986); Ogier, M. (1981) 'A study of the leadership style and verbal interactions of ward sisters and nurse learners', Unpublished Ph.D Thesis, London, Birkbeck College.
5 RCN (1978b), p. 54.
6 Gibberd, F.B. (1983) 'The nursing career structure as seen by a hospital doctor', *British Medical Journal*, 12 March, 286, p. 913.
7 Clark, M.O. (1984) *in* Duncan and McLachlan (eds), p. 51.
8 Mackay, L. and Torrington, D. (1986) 'Training in the UK: down but not out', *Journal of European Industrial Training*, 10, 1, p. 11–16.
9 RCN (1978b), p. 53.
10 Salvage (1985), p. 21.
11 DHSS (1972), p. 19.

12 See Cousins (1987), p. 103.
13 See Batchelor, I. (1984) Contrast between the professions' *in* Duncan and McLachlan (eds) *Hospital Medicine and Nursing in the 1980s: Interaction Between the Professions of Medicine and Nursing*, London, Nuffield Provincial Hospitals Trust. p. 76.
14 ACAS *in* Merrison (1979), p. 460.
15 Cousins (1987), p. 171.
16 There was a rapid growth in trade union membership in the NHS in the 1970s which corresponded with the changes in management – see Carpenter (1982) 'The labour movement in the National Health Service (NHS): UK' *in* Sethi, A.S. and Dimmock, S. (eds) *Industrial Relations and Health Services*, London, Croom Helm, p. 72.
17 See also Carpenter *in* Sethi and Dimmock (eds) (1982).
18 See ACAS *in* Merrison (1979), p. 464.
19 Salvage (1985), p. 20.
20 Salvage (1985), p. 61.
21 Salvage (1985), p. 97.
22 Cousins (1987), p. 188.
23 See Carpenter *in* Sethi and Dimmock (eds) (1982), p. 74.
24 See Carpenter *in* Sethi and Dimmock (eds) (1982), p. 85.
25 Brindle, D. (1988a) 'RCN keeps no strike line', *The Guardian*, 29 March.

9

Why Do They Do it?

Despite the many and varied demands made of nurses, most continue to derive a great deal of satisfaction from their jobs. There are good and bad, rewarding and frustrating patients. But the main source of satisfaction for nurses comes from their patients and in helping them. Nevertheless a large proportion of nurses felt they might leave in the following year. And a substantial minority would not choose nursing again. Yet many nurses obviously take pride in being a nurse. It can be a challenging and rewarding job. It is a worthwhile job in which women in particular can realize their potential. Nursing changes people: it increases their confidence but it can also make them 'harder' with regard to the less serious health complaints of relatives and friends. Thus nurses in keeping a smile on their face for patients are taken to task for not being caring enough at home. It seems that as women they can't win!

Nursing is a difficult job. It is a demanding and often stressful job. The policymakers and planners may want to know why nurses leave, but a more realistic perspective is why do they stay? Most of us say, and quite firmly too, that we would not or could not be a nurse. What do these nurses get from their jobs? Why do they do it?

Not surprisingly, different nurses find different satisfactions (as they find different dissatisfactions) in their work. For the most part, it's the patients who make the job. But the rewards from the patients come from a variety of aspects. It is not just life-saving activities, although they matter; satisfaction also comes from mundane things like making someone comfortable, getting a patient to smile or just seeing someone walk out of the ward.

> The patients. On a good day when they respond. After 2 years and they get your name right, it's fantastic . . . They all ate with

spoons in here when I came on in the beginning of January, and now they all use a knife and fork. (Staff Nurse)

I enjoy it, sometimes I'm fed up, but on the whole when you nurse somebody, especially down here when they are really ill and then you see them when they are getting better and then they go on to the wards and then they come back down and see us before they go home, really well, it's good. (Staff Nurse)

It's just the patients, I love the patients. It's not that I feel . . . I don't feel sorry for them, I don't feel like I'm here to change their lives. Just to be here to make it a bit easier, a bit more comfortable. (Enrolled Nurse)

I feel it's something worth while that I'm doing. And you do get rewards, hopefully seeing patients get well and going home or if its a terminal patient, helping them to face death or make the death as easy as possible. I feel that it's something worth while. (Sister)

It gives me a great deal of satisfaction actually. Seeing somebody comfortable and a nice smile and the relatives calm – I feel I'm doing some good. I like being good! (District Nurse)

I think it's the satisfaction of helping people really. You know, working with people and knowing maybe that you've helped them a little bit. It isn't always Florence Nightingale mopping the fevered brow lark, you know, it's just working with people, knowing you've helped them. (Student)

Quite a number of the nurses' comments focus on their role as defenders of the patients, making sure that they are given the best especially when they are helpless.

Client contact, the knowing you've actually, hopefully, changed somebody's life for the better and given them the opportunities that I had without having to demand them. They are a group of people that can't demand for themselves, they can't be vocal, so somebody has to do it and somebody has to make sure that they get what they deserve. (Sister)

I like helping people, I like people. I like to be around people, especially people who cannot do for themselves. You know, it's just knowing you've done your good deed for the day sort of thing . . . I just love the old people, I think they are super. You have got so much to learn from them, no matter how 'mental' they are, they still remember things that have happened in the past and you can talk to them. (Pupil)

There is a good deal of excitement to be found in nursing, in the unexpected and emergency situations when particular demands are placed on nurses.

> There were times at 3 o'clock in the morning if the 'phone rang and I thought, Oh God, its freezing, I don't know if I want to go but by the time I'd got dressed and I'd got out the adrenalin was going. I went to work and if we were lucky and we saved somebody's life you know, to come home and feel it was worth it. What was the loss of 4 hours' sleep, you'd done a good job and that to me made it worth while. (Staff Nurse)

> It's fun for me personally, it can be fun. At other times it's stimulating and that's quite good – There's one day they are lively and jovial and you can have a lot of fun with them, they are stimulating. Also, the violence I suppose – the bit of danger, you are uncertain what's happening, you've got to keep on top of that. And to top it all I think I'm doing a good turn or something, helping somebody. (Pupil)

> I like looking after people. I like feeling responsibility. I like delegating work. I like the feeling when everything's gone well at the end of the shift. I suppose all that. I like the sort of excitement when it's busy, yes, I get satisfaction out of that. (Staff Nurse)

The decision making and responsibility were remarked upon by quite a few nurses. For some of these nurses the satisfaction of their work was in realizing their own potential.

> I like the opportunities for making decisions. I like being able to use my own initiative; gaining knowledge and being able to use that knowledge. (Staff Nurse)

There are pleasures to be found in being part of a smoothly functioning team:

> When it flows nicely and the staff you are working with, the particular group are nice with you and you get a good camaraderie and everybody is working together and the surgeons are nice and the registrars. The sister is excellent where I am now. (Staff Nurse)

The satisfactions which these nurses refer to seem to come from two sources: actually helping people (patients and relatives) and 'doing a good deed'. There is an awareness amongst nurses, sometimes made explicit, that they are doing a job which others will not do. The special qualities required of nurses distinguishes them from others. A notion of vocation is involved as well. Although I did not ask nurses about their religious beliefs, the idea of having a vocation is similar to that expressed by those in religious orders. It is perhaps not a coincidence that nuns often engage in nursing work.

Nursing is different from other jobs. Most nurses have worked in other occupations and have some basis for comparison. For some, nursing is addictive:

> I've always wanted to be a nurse. I've always enjoyed it, I always will. I'm one of these that do moan because we are short-staffed but I will get on with it. It is very, very stressful at the moment, you do get very frustrated. But I don't know, I wouldn't do anything else. (Enrolled Nurse)

> It's something I've always enjoyed doing. Its the companionship, the feeling that you are doing something worth while. It's not just a job, it gets to be a way of life. And I think you get to be addicted to it. (Sister)

> . . . it's difficult to leave once you are into it – it sort of gets hold of you. I cannot imagine leaving it. (Enrolled Nurse)

But for a few nurses, the job had lost any satisfactions or rewards. As intrinsic satisfactions wane, extrinsic satisfactions such as money become important.[1] They may have been working in a specialty which they dislike or they may simply have been in nursing too long.

> I don't get anything out of nursing like I used to when I was training. I think you can stagnate . . . after you've been on a certain unit for a certain number of years, I think they should change it round so that you could go onto medical or surgical or children's and then rotate around so that you don't sort of stagnate in the same place. (Enrolled Nurse)

> I don't think I get as much out of it now to tell the truth, as I did out of general training because I don't feel – they are not ill to begin with, you don't feel you need to make them better. But I like being with people anyway, I like talking to people. (Student)

> I enjoy the patients and helping them . . . But I suppose to be honest I've stayed in it so long; half because I need the money and half because it is what I trained for. During my training I was always looking for other jobs. (Enrolled Nurse)

It was predominantly enrolled nurses who complained about the lack of satisfaction from their work. Enrolled nurses have extremely limited promotion prospects and it may be that the thought of doing the same work for the rest of their working lives, without any substantial change, is particularly daunting. Enrolled nurses may be less able to hang on to the idea of a vocation and thus, tend to see nursing in more instrumental terms. In other words, nursing becomes simply another job.

It is interesting that a few of the learners said they would complete their training because they had started it and wanted to have a qualification behind them. However, they felt that they would not continue in nursing once they had actually qualified. This may change as they progress into their second year of nursing if they find there is an 'addictive' element to the job, or the alternatives seem less possible:

> I still want to join the police force but I'm too small and they won't have me. I thought if I've got a qualification like nursing behind me it might sway them a bit on my height. (Clare)

> At the moment I'm saying that I will hopefully qualify in 3 years and then might leave nursing altogether and just use it as a qualification for something else, in psychiatry or just leave the nursing profession . . . I don't think I will carry on being a nurse. (Theresa)

Despite all the rewards that are to be found in nursing these are not always enough to make nurses stay, or want to stay where they are. Two-thirds of the stayers said in the questionnaire that they felt there was a chance they might leave in the next 12 months. The other third said there was definitely no chance they would be leaving the hospital in the next 12 months. Nearly half of the twenty-one learners I spoke to had considered leaving at some stage during their first year of training. Thoughts about leaving vary. Some nurses daydream in a desultory way about a different career while others are quite adamant that they do want to try something different.

> I don't know because I say I'd leave but whether I will . . . it sounds muddled up, but you get so used to nursing and . . . well, because you care and you want to care for other people . . . I will go one day and I will do something different. I will probably go back to college and study something that I want to do. (Enrolled Nurse)

> I've enjoyed it up to now but now I feel that I am definitely ready for a change. (Charge Nurse)

Complaints about aspects such as 'the hierarchy' or the lack of career prospects also caused nurses to think of leaving:

> The fact that I would leave nursing makes me angry because I

enjoy the job I do. If they would just leave us alone to do our job we'd be a lot happier. I'd miss it, I'd miss it an awful lot because I'm interested in the work I do. I've done quite a few nursing studies sort of things. But it's coming into conflict with the hierarchy makes you ask 'why do I put up with this?'. (Enrolled Nurse)

I'm 35 and I don't feel I want to be a ward Sister when I'm in my 40s, and I don't want to be a nursing officer. (Sister)

For others, there was little or no chance that they would leave nursing. The replies from these nurses were short and to the point! 'Not really . . . it's my life is nursing' (Enrolled Nurse). 'No, never' (Sister). So while many nurses did think about leaving, only a small minority were seriously considering it.[2] As in any other job, a bad day can make you think about trying something, anything, else. As nursing provides very stressful situations, it seems relatively easy to have a bad day.

However, despite the rewards of nursing and the rather half-hearted comments about leaving, some nurses feel trapped in the job. A third of the questionnaire nurses as well as those interviewed said they would not or they didn't know if they would still choose nursing if they were to go back to the beginning. A recurring theme was the lack of career advice given to young women in their final years at school. Both of the following comments were made by nurses in their early 30s. It is, therefore, not that long ago since they chose their career. It seems unlikely that the quality of career advice for young women has much improved.

I did nursing because it ran in the family: my mother was a nurse, a cousin, an auntie. I don't think I had enough career information while I was at school. I think really teaching I would have enjoyed. (Staff Nurse)

If I knew then what I know now, no. No way . . . I was really pressurized when I was 18 'what are you going to do?', so it was I'll be a nurse because I didn't want to go to teachers' training and the options were you either went into a bank, did teachers' training or you became a nurse. (Sister)

The actual experience of nursing was what might deter others from choosing to do nursing again.

I don't think I would. I think I'd try and do something else. Something a bit less stressful. Perhaps a bit easier really. I mean, it is damned hard work. (Enrolled Nurse)

Oh no, no way and when I see these first years coming in now I
just feel like screaming at them 'don't do it, go and do something
else'. You know, we look at first years sometimes and the
comments that come out from nurses: 'they must be mad'; 'if
only they knew what they were letting themselves in for'. (Staff
Nurse)

However, the majority of nurses said they would still choose nursing.[3]
Their comments show that they are not always starry-eyed about it.

I don't know. I'm proud of what I've achieved to get to a ward
sister. When I started out I never thought in a million years I
would ever be ward sister. But then it's not all it's cracked up to
be. Everybody thinks: 'Oh, a ward sister, she's doing all right' but
sometimes I think it's not worth it, it's not worth the hassle.
(Sister)

If I had to start again, yes, but now I don't think I would advise
my daughter to go into nursing . . . I did get a lot of job
satisfaction but there seems to be a lot of stress . . . I would not
say, no, but I would not encourage her. (District Nurse)

Mmm, that's something I've asked myself many times and I just
don't know the answer! I think it's been a very interesting life
certainly and it does have a lot of rewards but it is quite a tough
life . . . And I think at some of the more distressing times it
started to impinge on my personal life and my home life . . . it
gets on top of you. But whether I would have wanted to avoid all
that I don't know, because it's been a very enriching experience.
(Health Visitor)

Given the stresses and strains which seems to be inherent in so much
of nursing work it would be unreasonable to expect unmitigated
enthusiasm for the job. But even though many nurses have reservations about the work they do, it also provides rewards. Indeed, part of
the reward may be the overcoming of the bad days and the negative
experiences by the good days and the successes. Nevertheless, there
are quite a number of nurses who, unreservedly, enjoy their jobs and
would have no hesitation in choosing it again.

Yes, I'm sorry I didn't do it when I was younger. This is definitely
my vocation – I should have seen it sooner. (Enrolled Nurse)

Yes, I have been very happy doing it, and I do enjoy coming to
work. I love the patients; I seem to be able to communicate with
them, and I think if you've got somebody who wants some
help . . . at the end of the day, I know it sounds a bit corny, but I
do enjoy it. (Sister)

Yes, I don't regret coming into nursing at all. It's opened my eyes to a great many things. The way other people live, the problems other people have to contend with, people's behaviours . . . (Staff Nurse)

Nursing does have a substantial impact on those who take it up. I asked both qualified nurses and the learners, whether they felt that they had been changed by nursing. The answer was a resounding *Yes*.

For some nurses, however, the question was impossible to answer. Rather on the lines of asking if the medicine has done any good: 'I don't know how I would have turned out otherwise!' (Sister). Similarly, for those nurses who had been older when they first started their training, they were less likely to be dramatically affected by their nursing experience. Even so, one pupil who was older – in her mid-twenties – when she started her training felt that: 'I think I am becoming my own person more and not just a Mum at home' (Sheila). Other nurses reported that they had also experienced an increase in their own self-esteem:

It's given me a lot of skills that I never had . . . and I think it's given me a feeling of self worth I think . . . And I think I'm doing something socially useful at the end of the day. (Charge Nurse)

As will be seen below, a growth in confidence and self-esteem seems to happen fairly often when working as a nurse.

The most frequently mentioned change was a more tolerant attitude and a greater awareness of the problems of others.

It has certainly made me more understanding . . . but I think it perhaps made me more humble, seeing how so many people suffer and also the problems that people have. You see other people's lives in a totally different light. (District Nurse)

Yes, I used to be very self-centred, now I am only moderately self-centred! (Enrolled Nurse)

It's made me more aware of people's problems. I used to tend to walk around with my head in the clouds. But here you can't. Homelessness, lack of funds, lack of care. Some of them don't really need to come into hospital, it's only a breakdown in community care which has brought them back, and things like that. (Staff Nurse)

An increase in confidence and a reduction in shyness were aspects which were to be mentioned again and again. Of course, many of these nurses went into the job when they were fairly young and it is only to be expected that they would experience a rise in confidence as they grew older. However, there seems little doubt that nursing can speed up the process.

> It is probably because I got older as well. I came straight into nursing. I have become quite confident, I am still quite a shy person but I have become more self-assertive. Sometimes I think you have to be to survive. (Staff Nurse)

> Yes, I think you become more adult . . . from the beginning, I'm thinking as an 18-year-old, you grow up much more quickly than an 18-year-old would have done and I think you keep that maturity ahead of yourself all of the time. (Sister)

Learners have to grow up quickly. Field, for example, notes 'the care of the dying often devolves to the untrained and training nurses . . . who are unskilled, unprepared and often unsupported'.[4] Nurse learners have, after all, a far harsher introduction to suffering than medical students.[5] Medical students and doctors are physically and emotionally more remote from patients than nurses.[6] For nurses sitting holding the hand of a dying patient it is not easy to be emotionally remote. It means growing up quickly. The strains of coming to terms with so many different experiences and situations were apparent from comments from learners:

> Here you go to work under pressure, you come back under pressure and you feel like you are getting so many wrinkles. You are weighed down by pressure. By the time we qualify we will be old women. It does that, it takes all your youth away from you because they expect you to grow up so much. (Julie)

Part of the process of gaining in confidence is becoming more assertive and being able to speak up for yourself.

> Well I wouldn't say boo to a goose before, you know. I mean I was very frightened. I've got more confidence now than I did before. And I'm not frightened to walk in front of people and just ask a question or whatever I want. I wouldn't do that at one time, so it's built up my confidence that way and I'm not as shocked as I used to be – I mean especially in a place like this . . . the swearwords that come out . . . at first I just couldn't get used to it, but I'm not so shocked any more really. (Pupil)

> I think so because it broadens your personality an awful lot. I was quite shy and quiet when I first came into nursing but it certainly doesn't pay to be like that. I certainly don't think you could survive in the nursing structure if you were. I wouldn't say it was a bad change because I think it makes a better person of you. (Staff Nurse)

There was a change, seldom seen as positive, that of becoming harder.[7] Many of the nurses who felt that they had become harder obviously regretted the change in themselves. There were repercussions as far as their families were concerned as well. This 'hardness' seemed to vary from person to person. For some, the hardness was a smokescreen, disguising their vulnerability.

> You get used to certain things, you know. Things don't tend to shock you the same, as they would before, but that doesn't mean you've become harder because you still get hurt the same. (Student)

Some felt they had become hard with regard to the ailments of their friends and families while retaining great sympathy for their patients. The 'hardness' at times really seems to be more of a bitterness that some patients suffered a great deal. Coping with the 'unfair deaths' of children, young adults, parents of young families must make everyday ailments very much into irrelevancies.

> the patients you see . . . who are really poorly and the terminally ill and the small babies that are poorly with leukaemia . . . I got really involved with them and I was very sympathetic and . . . it upset me, very much so. Of course when you go home and your father is complaining of a cold and this sort of thing, that's what I mean by not being – so it's hardened me that way. (Staff Nurse)

> I think I am hard now. It doesn't take a lot for me to snap at somebody. I snap at my daughter a lot and I know I shouldn't. If she's ill or my husband's ill, they don't get sympathy. I'll say 'go up there and look at some of those in the beds' but I don't get any sympathy in return, so it comes back to me. (Sister)

Some nurses said they had become 'cynical' when they talked about becoming hardened. This seemed to be a reflection of the judgement of friends outside nursing who expect a nurse to be compassionate, sympathetic and constantly caring. One or two nurses obviously felt hard and lacking in compassion towards patients. But for the others, their badge of cynicism was worn with resignation. Resignation perhaps at being misunderstood, because it was clear that they still cared for and were compassionate towards their patients.

> Yes it does. I have become very cynical and hard. Yes, I would say so. I have become very critical. If you are really tired at night it alters things in your personal life – also, doing nights . . . (Staff Nurse)

> I'm cynical, very cynical these days. People outside say I'm not very sympathetic, when somebody is ill, it's nothing, I brush it

off. And they expect you to come across as this compassionate
sympathetic person and I'm not at all . . . You give out so much
at work that you like to think in your leisure time that . . . you
can't continually, 24 hours a day, 7 days a week, give all the
time. (Sister)

But it should not be surprising if some nurses, having to deal with so
many deaths, so many terminally ill patients, having to help people
who will not help themselves, facing the problems that society wants
to sweep under the carpet, do become harder. For the most part,
nurses have to look in the face the hard facts of life which most of us
want to turn away from. If a nurse has drifted into nursing rather
than believing she or he has a vocation, it may mean they have less
armour to shield themselves against the harsh realities of caring.
When nursing is felt to be a vocation or a lifelong dream, then those
harsh realities may be more easily accepted as a part of their chosen
occupation.

In looking at how nurses become changed by nursing, one essential
element, the patient, should not be overlooked. At the start of this
chapter the centrality of patients to the rewards which nurses often
get from their jobs was quite apparent. However, 'the patient' isn't
always the nice, kind, appreciative and passive recipient of care.
Patients come in all sorts of packages. Some are kind, some are tetchy.
Some are helpful, some obstructive. Some are likeable, others are
anything but.

Qualified nurses rarely mention the specific idiosyncrasies of
patients. It may be, as Salvage suggests, that 'there is pressure to get
on with all the patients'.[8] Or nurses may have become accustomed to
the variety and the vagaries of the patients. The patients become an
accepted part of the job. The learners, however, were in the process of
finding out about patients: they had not yet become accustomed to
them. As a result, learners often made comments about the patients,
making explicit what qualified nurses may take for granted.

In the first place, some patients are nicer and easier to relate to than
others. It is not surprising that when nurses do have a spare moment
they choose to talk to someone they like.

Some patients you'll find you go and talk to but it's normally the
ones that you get on with better. You find you'll find minutes to
sit and talk with them or just stand and talk with them. I think
it's something you can't help: you tend to go towards people who
appeal to you! (Alice)

It is quite clear that, no matter where they are, nurses will like some
patients a good deal less than others.

There are the odd ones you get attached to. Not so much attached, you get on with well. But they come and go. (Mary)

. . . some people do try your patience. I think you've got to be patient with your patients. I think you learn to control your patience with people. You know, show them one thing when you are thinking: 'Oh, go away.' (Kay)

Some people are able and they just let you do everything for them which I don't like really. (Dorothy)

I think there's only been one I didn't like – on male surgical. This fellow was disgusting – he never washed himself or cleaned up after himself. His room, he was in a side room, it was absolutely filthy. (Susan)

Learning not to show your feelings is a very important part of becoming a nurse. Menzies comments that 'there is almost an explicit "ethic" that any patient must be treated the same as any other patient'.[9] It is necessary to disguise feelings of dislike about any patient. The fact that patients can be unlikeable and rude was seldom raised by the qualified nurses. Salvage comments on this fact as well: 'no attempt is made to talk about the anger or resentment which nurses feel towards particular patients . . .'.[10,11] The learners, on the other hand, were still in the process of learning how to cope with unlikeable patients and many comments about such patients were made.

And it's hard to sort of keep a smile on your face all the time, sort of being *pleasant* to everybody because some of the patients can be nasty as well. They just take you for granted half the time. (Dorothy)

We've got one patient on there and he shouts at everybody – he just wants attention. And there are times, especially when you're rushed off your feet and you sort of think 'if he shouts once more, I'll . . .' and you walk in with your hands behind your back and say 'Yes, Frank, what do you want?' – but he does the same with everybody. (Sheila)

you can't say you like every patient that you treat but you can't show that you don't like them. (Clare)

Perhaps even more important is the necessity to conceal any disgust that might be felt in nursing a patient. Nurses have to carry out extremely intimate tasks which may be embarrassing for the patient. A nurse must appear impassive to tasks which the patients themselves find distressing.

Colostomies – I'm not so keen on. The smell is unbelievable. It's not from what comes out, it's just the smell. The patients are so embarrassed you have to pretend that you can't smell anything. I just say I've got a permanently blocked nose – you can't let them know that it does bother you. (Alice)

Similarly nurses have the problem of coping with the questions of dying patients. Some patients may be told they are dying but not how long they have to live. Other patients may not be told they are dying. At the same time, the relatives of patients may not be informed of the patient's prognosis. The decisions not to divulge information may be taken by members of the medical profession but it is nurses on whom the burden of concealment falls. In other words, the nurse acts as a buffer between the professional and the layman.[12] Nurses may not like the fact that a patient is not being informed of her or his impending death, but nevertheless they must go along with the opinion of the doctor. Concealment of the diagnosed state of health of a patient is a skill which nurses must learn. When learners first go on to a ward they can, in the face of a patient's questions, plead ignorance, e.g. 'I am not given that sort of information'. As the learners progress through their first allocations they must become accustomed to 'fielding' patients' searching questions. It is not easy.

I think the worst thing is just actually being asked – it's not when that person is actually dead, coping with that, it's before when they're going through all the agony 'Am I going to die?' and maybe you've been told that they're not supposed to know and that situation I find quite distressing. (Ann)

Also not easy is learning that the attitude of some qualified nurses towards the patients, may leave something to be desired. Indeed, the learners were sometimes shocked by some of the practices and attitudes they encountered.

People, when you're not in nursing, don't always expect that nurses are human beings I suppose, and they expect you to always like, well not necessarily like all the patients but not to be funny with them. And I think you find a lot of nurses' attitudes to patients are rotten. And the way they talk to them and about them . . . Somebody can explain a better way for the patient to do things but they won't do the things that are better for them. They do what they like, routine or anything, rather than what is better for the patients, like just slap 'em down in chairs sort of thing. That's one of the biggest disappointments. (Alice)

. . . there's not a happy atmosphere on most of the wards, you can't have chats with your patients. The patients aren't really happy and they don't like asking you for things because they can see that you are too busy. There's nurses that are just so inconsiderate, like putting meals at the bottom of people's beds that they know just can't reach them. (Julie)

The number of specific instances in which the attitudes of qualified staff towards patients come in for criticism from the learners was not high. However, the fact that there were such occasions – and some of them were quite serious – when the attitudes and behaviour of qualified staff left a great deal to be desired, added to the disillusioning of the learners. It must also contribute towards making new recruits 'harder' and more cynical.[13] Learners are constantly being watched by the patients as well as being supervised and monitored by qualified staff. They have to learn that they are 'on display' all the time and to behave accordingly.

the patients take their lead from the way the staff behave and how they behave to each other because they listen and watch everything you say to each other and about each other. You couldn't have any secrets. THEY know, you could ask them which nurses like which nurses, because they've nothing else to do all day but sit there and watch you a lot of the time. (Alice)

Some patients play up to the fact that nurses are 'on display' and ensure that the maximum publicity is given to them. The learners have to learn to ignore some patients' attempts at amateur dramatics and to get on with the job in hand.

There was one patient, she had got bad legs but she needed to get the circulation going. We wanted to get her to the bathroom and she was screaming: 'How can you be so cruel.' (Laura)

At the same time, learners find out that their patients do not simply exist in the clean and warm hospital. Those neat and tidy patients in a hospital ward can be found to be living in poverty and squalor. Thus, exposure to nursing in the community can be an eye-opener:

I think you realize how better off you are. I didn't think people lived in such . . . you know, some of the places are a bit grim. I didn't realize people lived in places like that, really dirty and cold. I've never really been into places like that so it's been an eye-opener. I've never seen anything like that before. When you're in hospital all the time, somebody comes in and maybe their clothes are a bit dirty, you know, but you don't really know until you go into their houses and see . . . (Barbara)

While the learners make reappraisals of their perception of nurses and of patients, they also develop expectations about how patients *ought* to behave. The learners start to make their own definitions of what constitutes a 'good' or a 'bad' patient.

> The worst thing is people who don't say 'thank you'. They just go. I know a lot of them are just glad to get out, I think I would be if I was a patient, but it's really nice when people take the time to say it. (Kay)

> Some patients are really . . . they don't say please or thank you. I have a bad habit of saying 'thank-you' when I give out a cup of tea or something. I think some patients think I'm trying to be cheeky. But I'm not, it just comes out naturally! (Wendy)

Many judgements as to 'good' or 'bad' patients appear to be related to gender. Half of the learners clearly preferred to nurse males.[14] Only three learners preferred to nurse females. The other learners didn't have any preferences as to the gender of their patients. It is interesting to consider some of their comments because they illustrate the expectations which exist within nursing about the behaviour of patients. For example, the 'good' patient should not complain.

> Oh the females are always wingeing – they're not bad you know but it's just . . . the males are more get up and do things for themselves, they are easier to push along. (Susan)

And the 'good' patient should try to help the nurses and not let the nurses run around after them.

> One went home yesterday – he kept pressing his buzzer every 5 minutes. Sister normally sorts him out, she normally goes down and sorts him out! They don't take much notice of you when they know you're a student: if you tell them to stop doing things, they don't respect you as much . . . (Kay)

> When I was on male surgical I enjoyed that because the men tried to . . . they DID help, which was quite amazing really. But the women just sort of thought: 'Oh, I'm in hospital, I'll have a holiday, and let everybody run after me' instead of them running after everyone else which is fair enough. I don't blame them in one respect but it makes our life hard work. (Dorothy)

> I enjoy nursing them both really. I think you can have a bit more fun with males, they tend to be a bit less serious with themselves, they tend to be a bit more jovial and you can jolly them along a bit. (Heather)

What is so intriguing is that men are often said to be poor invalids when they are at home. They are popularly held to complain a great deal and feel very sorry for themselves. Women on the other hand, who are not well at home tend to have to keep going and not to give in. It seems that when they get to hospital, women gratefully give in to all the ministrations that are available. Men, on the other hand, while they may be prepared to be real invalids at home, dislike the helplessness and lack of control they face in hospital. Helpless in the face of the (mainly) young women who briskly order them about and tell them what to do, the men may react by distancing themselves as soon as possible from this state. The women don't complain at home, the men do. The men don't complain in hospital, the women do. Nurses prefer to nurse men rather than women. This is an obvious simplification and over-generalization. Nevertheless, out of the learners who did express a preference, three-quarters chose males. Even though some of the learners appreciated the situation in which women found themselves, their preference was still for nursing men.

However, those that expressed no preference, pointed to both negative and positive aspects of either gender. The attribute which was valued in dealing with women was that they were easier to relate to:

But I find it easier I think to sit down and talk to a female if they're really distressed – both have got their advantages. (Heather)

Whether it's just because I started on a female ward first, I don't know. I enjoy both but I find I do tend to get more feedback from female. (Mary)

It is not at all clear that feminism has had much influence amongst the recruits to nursing. But one or two learners did mention factors such as 'the oppression of women' and they were obviously aware of, at least some, social, domestic, and economic factors which affected women's lives.

Not all nurses equally value the contact with patients. Some prefer to work in environments where patient-contact is limited such as in Theatre. As the learners progress through their training their preferences regarding patient contact crystallize:

No I don't miss the patient-contact that much. Because you can have a good talk with the surgeons – it becomes more technical than nursing-wise, mopping the brow . . . (Clare)

You don't actually get to know your patients, it's a very quick turnover. You just see them for a few minutes and then are asleep and they go back to the wards. (Eileen)

I just really enjoyed it [recovery] – it's total patient care, you've got to be with them all the time, you've got to be watching them all the time, and it's one-to-one all the time. You're not sort of running round thinking: 'Oh God, who have I got to see next?' (Julie)

For those learners who do seek patient-contact, the relationship which nurses can have with patients varies from specialty to specialty. In some areas, patients are only in hospital for a short stay. Elsewhere as in medicine for the elderly, mental illness and mental handicap, the patients are often in hospital or a hostel for a considerable time. Some nurses relish the thought of building long-term relationships and where there is often no obvious improvement in the patient's condition. But for other nurses, the rewards of the job are in a speedy turnover of patients where results are more immediate.

In surgical, because they're in and they're out you don't get much of a chance to get a relationship going with a patient very well. (Ann)

In medical you get to know them [the patients] . . . but also I think it can get a bit monotonous. If you are seeing different faces, younger people, older people, you've got more variety. (Dorothy)

In the medical ward they're all sort of elderly patients and that was more upsetting and very hard work. But I liked surgical ward because they were sort of coming in and out very quickly, you saw people get better and go home. (Sally)

This preference for the 'speedy turnover' of the surgical wards illustrates the way in which the medical profession's priorities can be adopted, almost unnoticed, by nurses. This finding should not occasion surprise. After all, the NHS as a whole is dominated by the concept of cure and the acute sector as its fulcrum.[15] For those nurses working outside the general hospital environment, there are different relationships with patients. For mental patients who may have been in a hospital for decades, the fleeting visits of students may make little impact on their everyday lives. After all, the hospital is their home and the learners who come and go are simply visitors who are not always welcome. But for some students, working in a mental hospital was rewarding:

I've really enjoyed it here [in a long stay rehabilitation ward] – it's very different. I'd like to stay here another 18 months and qualify and get a job here . . . The patients are more rewarding here than in general [nursing]. (Theresa)

For other learners, and they were in the majority, nursing in psychiatry was neither enjoyable nor rewarding. Indeed, quite a number of the students found the experience threatening.

> I find it quite stressful . . . it's more relaxed but some of the ladies, their moods swing a lot – they've got schizophrenia and . . .And I can't predict what their mood is going to be and I find it quite nerve-wracking that they might turn round and give me a whack or something. (Ann)

There is a different kind of challenge in working within the community. The clients are on home ground whereas in hospital, patients are on someone else's territory. The relationship between nurse and patient is obviously affected. At home the clients cannot be told what to do, they can only be advised. In other words, the authority of the nurse changes.

> It [community] is really good – it's different . . . They're different at home to what they are in hospital so you get to see both sides. It's their house and they're in charge. Some will say, you know, 'the nurse is here' and run and fetch for the nurse, but for a lot of them it's their house and you're a guest in their house which alters it slightly. (Wendy)

As the experiences of the learners demonstrate, there are many different environments and types of relationships which come under the banner of 'nursing'. When nurses say their satisfaction comes from the patients, they mean many different things. Some mean the relationships they build up, while others mean the number of patients they have helped. Nursing covers such a range of activities that it does some injustice to the individuals who are working as nurses to lump them all together. Midwives or qualified nurses who care for the mentally handicapped often point out that they are not 'nurses' or that they do not do a nursing job. It has been argued, for example, that health visitors have to 'unlearn' their past as nurses before they can become successful health visitors.[16] Working with the mentally handicapped may primarily involve teaching rather than 'nursing'. There are nurses who are technically expert in intensive care, or working in operating theatres who do work which is very different from the nurses who work in the general wards. Nevertheless, running through the accounts of the nurses from these disparate groups is the importance of the patient. It is for the benefit of patients that many nurses feel they nurse.

The idea of doing a worthwhile job is obviously important to many nurses. Whether esteem is in one's own eyes or in the eyes of the

world, it acts to keep nurses nursing. Nurses have come through the
often traumatic process of learning to be a nurse. They have survived
the trials of training and they have met the demands placed upon
them. There is not a little pride in such an accomplishment. While
their initial enthusiasms may be dampened their commitment to
nursing may have increased. Nurses may have a commitment to
nursing because they have invested so much time and effort in
becoming qualified or because they have invested their own self-
concept in their chosen career. The idea of having a vocation protects
some nurses from the frustrations and difficulties of working as a
nurse. For others, nursing is addictive, a job they have learned to love
despite all its negative aspects. What makes the job worth while for
most of these nurses is the patient. The various difficulties encountered in nursing are not yet sufficient to counter the rewards that
nurses obtain from their patients. That is why nurses stay.

Notes

1 Orientations to work are discussed fully in Goldthorpe, J.H., Lockwood,
   D., Bechhofer, F. and Platt, J. (1968) and Daniel (1969).
2 In DHSS (1972) only a very small proportion of hospital nurses – only 3
   per cent – thought they would be working outside nursing in two years'
   time, p. 18.
3 A similar finding was made by West and Rushton (1986), p. 30.
4 Field, D. (1984) '"We didn't want him to die on his own" – nurses'
   accounts of nursing dying patients', *Journal of Advanced Nursing*, 9, p. 60.
5 Muir Gray (1980), p. 22.
6 Muir Gray (1980), p. 22.
7 A process that Menzies has described as a 'defensive psychological
   detachment' (1970), p. 28.
8 Salvage (1985), p. 66.
9 Menzies 1970, p. 14.
10 Salvage (1985), p. 66.
11 An examination of these issues is made by Menzies (1970).
12 Dolan (1987), p. 10.
13 The need for nurses to accept occasional patient abuse, or leave, has been
   explored by Stannard, C. (1975) 'Old folks and dirty work: the social
   conditions for patient abuse in a nursing home' *in* Dingwall and McIntosh
   (eds), Chapter 11.
14 This runs contrary to Menzies belief that qualified nurses find it difficult to
   express preferences regarding types of patients or about gender of
   patients, and suggests that only partial socialization of learners regarding
   the 'good' patient has taken place – (1970), p. 12.
15 See Clark, J. (1979) 'The British National Health Service 1948–1978:
   should we start again?', *Journal of Advanced Nursing*, 4, p. 209.
16 McIntosh, J. and Dingwall, R. (1978) 'Teamwork in theory and practice'
   in Dingwall and McIntosh, p. 128.

10

The 'Good Nurse'

Underlying many of the actions and beliefs of nurses is their ideal type of nurse: the good nurse. There appears to be broad agreement from those at the top and those just entering nursing on the attributes of the 'good nurse'. Commitment, character and caring are necessary attributes – skill is not mentioned. Because nursing is what women do naturally, then the equating of nursing with skilled work is unnecessary. At the same time, in seeking recognition for the skills involved, there has been a move to seek professional status for nursing. This move potentially poses threats to other members of the health care team. Nevertheless, the pursuit of professionalism is élitist and exclusive. In particular it will act so as to divide a female occupation into one group of highly paid and skilled qualified nurses and another group comprizing all the other women who undertake caring work. It must be asked then, who benefits if nurses seek to professionalize their occupation?

Running through the accounts of nurses' experiences, their moans and their satisfactions is an implicit idea of the 'good nurse'. This idea serves as a benchmark for their own and other nurses' behaviour and standards while nursing. For each nurse and for each patient what constitutes a 'good nurse' is slightly different.[1] Nevertheless, there are common threads running through many of the nurses' accounts as to definitions of the good nurse.

In the next chapter it will be seen that there is a relative lack of concern amongst the nurses as to whether they work in the private or the NHS. This lack of concern should not really cause any surprise. Nursing is attractive, as we have seen, for many reasons. But one of the most pervading reasons is nurses' wish to care for, and be caring of, patients. No judgement of the patient is made. Whether the patient is a Hindi or a Quaker is irrelevant to the good nurse. Whether the patient is paying directly or indirectly for treatment is also irrelevant. And, whether the nurse likes or dislikes the patient should also be irrelevant to the good nurse.

What is a 'good nurse'? What is the ideal state to which learners aspire? In the first place, the notion of a 'good nurse' is formed as the result of many different experiences and expectations. Common-sense notions are overlaid with personal experiences and the stereotyped views of the nurse from the mass media.[2] For the recruits to nursing, the view of what constitutes a 'good nurse' changes as they proceed through their training and see nurses nursing at first hand. At the end of their first year, the pupils and students were asked what qualities made a good nurse. The seven nursing officers were also asked what they felt made a good nurse. There is surprisingly little difference between the two groups.

Being aware of, and attuned to, the needs of patients was the frequently mentioned attribute of the 'good nurse'. Nurses also ought to be patient and compassionate, to be thoughtful and to be easy-going.[3] The learners said a good nurse should be intelligent, confident, and with what might be called good interpersonal skills.

> You have got to be understanding. You have got to care but you have not got to let your emotions run away with you. You have got to control yourself. You have got to be able to cope with other people's problems. I think the main thing is getting on with other staff because flipping heck, you don't half get some name-calling as soon as someone is out of the room! (Sheila)

It is interesting that it was particularly the students who mentioned the need for intelligence. Maybe this is a reflection of the greater number of O and A levels required from them compared with the pupil nurses.

> . . . you need to be intelligent, caring. You need to be conscious of the problem and you need to be able to cope with any problems. You need to understand your patient . . . That's what makes a good nurse: instead of telling someone to go and do that, you need to be prepared to do it yourself. (Eileen)

> You've just got to want to be part of a team that is doing something for somebody else. You know, to be able to just feel pleased with yourself when something goes right and grit your teeth and bear it when it doesn't. Just to be somebody that wants to do something for somebody else – nothing in particular. (Yvonne)

They've got to be caring. They've got to be a good listener because these patients do want to talk to you. They do, at times, want to tell us their problems – something is bothering them and they've got to have somebody that they can say it to. You've got to care about other people and want to help other people, I think too, to make a good nurse. (Nursing Officer)

A few learners replied in terms of what a nurse ought NOT to be. As we saw in Chapter 6, the 'good nurse' ought not to be overly concerned with pay. And, while the good nurse needs to 'get on' with everyone: other nurses, colleagues, and patients, particularly negative qualities are bad temper, abrasiveness, and a lack of sympathy.

I don't like to see if somebody is in a bad mood, they come in in the morning and take it out on other staff and the patients – people shouldn't do that because we are professionals and we should act like it. It upsets the patients . . . (Susan)

Well I see a good nurse as someone who sort of thinks about everything about the patient . . . Ones that are kind will sit and listen if they can [to the patients] – not ones that are shouting or telling them off. You come across people, someone who has wet their bed, incontinent, it was an accident, they couldn't help it – and it's: 'Why have you done this again, you did it yesterday?' shouting at them and it puts a barrier up between you and the patient. One who is interested in the patient as a person and one who works on the ward and just doesn't sit down fagging in the linen cupboard or whatever. (Laura)

Other learners referred to the need for them to change as a result of entering nursing.

Good tempered – all the things I was not before I came into nursing! Patient, caring – I think they have to give part of themselves when necessary, like to their dying patients – they have got to give an extra bit of love really. (Patricia)

What is missing from these accounts of the 'good nurse' is any reference to expertise or skill.[4] Such an omission points to the continuing influence of the Nightingale emphasis on the character rather than on the skills of nurses.[5] It may also indicate that nurses give less attention to competence than they give to being a 'nice' person.

By the end of their first year, the learners seemed to know what was expected of them and the picture they held of the good nurse was what nursing officers would agree with. In other words, the socialization of these learners in this respect seems to take place with great efficacy.

Implicit and explicit in some of the comments about what makes a 'good nurse' is the belief that in order to nurse well, commitment is necessary. In other words, nursing is not an easy job. It is a job which on some days is quite hard to take. If you don't have that 'commitment' then you may just as well go.

> She has to want to be a nurse, she's really got to . . . and she's got to realize that its hard work both physically and mentally. They've got to be able to cope . . . I think we perhaps give young nurses too much responsibility . . . even at 21 it's an awful responsibility to be responsible for thirty people, ill people . . . (Nursing Officer)

Some learners already see nursing in terms of a vocation.

> I think it's something that you've really got to want to do. I don't think its a job that you can do just as a job. I mean there are so many things that could really get you down if you let them. (Yvonne)

Other learners were not so sure: they seemed to feel that the qualities of a good nurse could be acquired.

> They've got to be intelligent. Have a lot of common sense, a lot of initiative and confidence, and you need interpersonal skills – but there's nothing that you can't learn I don't think. (Heather)

For these learners nursing was a job which may still be different from other jobs but it is not tremendously different. The skills and attributes of a good nurse can be learned. By extension, the greater the amount of training, the higher the level of skills. Following this line of argument, nursing is not a 'vocation' into which individuals are born. In other words, taking up nursing is a conscious choice rather than a sort of instinctive impulse to care. In contrast, it is worth noting that the general belief is that it is women, for the most part, who are born with a 'vocation' for nursing. At least, only a small minority of nurses are men.

There is a continuing debate within nursing as to whether it is a vocation or whether it can aspire towards becoming a profession. It is a debate which has been aired through the proposals of the UKCC on their report *Project 2000*. This report, which recommends a fundamental change in the style and structure of nurse training, also envisages changes in the orientation of nursing (see Chapter 11.) For the moment, however, it needs to be borne in mind that there is this division within the ranks of nurses between the professionals and the vocationals. An integral part of the division concerns the very essence of nursing: is nursing a caring, loving, nurturing endeavour or is it a set of specialist skills carried out in a competent and professional manner? The answer of course is that nursing should be neither and it should be both. Nobody welcomes an ineffective but nice nurse. Nobody welcomes an efficient but distant nurse. What is wanted is a 'good nurse' – the kind, patient, intelligent, and caring nurse which the learners identify. But this nurse should also be competent and skilled. It appears that greater recognition of the amount of skill involved in nursing is required from those who do it (as was seen in the relationships between nurses in Chapter 7).

However, subsumed within the debate about 'professionalism' is the position of nurses with regard to other health care workers: to doctors, to social workers, to occupational therapists, etc. Nurses are not highly paid and they have been overtaken by some of the para-medical professions in recent years.[6] Nurses feel the public image of nurses differs from the reality and their own image of themselves.[7] The status and prestige of nursing do not appear to be rising. They are not falling in relation to the general public, but in terms relative to their para-medical colleagues they are losing ground. Part of the issue revolves round the fact that most nurses are women. The failure of nursing to be recognized as a profession in its own right is seen to be tied to the facts of gender. Nursing is women's work: a good woman is a good nurse.[8,9] The domination of women by men in so many spheres of activity: social, political, economic is echoed in nursing. There is a disproportionate number of men in the upper echelons of nursing. There is the recent introduction of a large number of male general managers at both district and regional health authority levels. They are positions which seem to require male qualities rather than the qualities of a female nurse according to Carpenter.[10] There is the domination of health care by the mainly male, medical profession. The need for a place in the sun for nurses has been expressed by many commentators. It is not clear that the road towards 'professionaliz-ation' is the way to achieve that place in the sun. To professionalize is to exclude those who are not qualified. It is élitist and it is essentially sexist because the unqualified health care workers who undertake nursing tasks are women. To professionalize means that a further division within the ranks of those who care for patients will be created. It would further distance nurses from the nursing and caring that is done by so many women for dependent relatives in their own homes. It would mean the existence of a highly specialized and élite group of nurses. It would also mean the existence, quite separately, of an inferior and very large group of unskilled women who act as carers. There would be a polarization between those who participate in the acute, high intervention worlds of medicine and those who work in the labour intensive, low intervention worlds of the elderly, the mentally ill and the handicapped. It would also allow a small workforce to be paid high salaries with another, larger group, being paid very low salaries. Nurses need to ask themselves the question as to whose interests would best be served if nursing were to become a profession.

Yet the attractions of professionalization for a workforce that is not given the respect it deserves from other members of the health care team cannot be denied. The fact that nursing is associated with women and with what women naturally do, denies the training and skill which nurses develop. It is not surprising that the feminist movement has been seen as influential in challenging the nurse's traditional role.[11] It is not possible to resolve here the debate on the professional versus vocational issue. At least if nursing cannot become a profession as such it can, as Salvage suggests, 'aspire to professionalism'.[12] The debate on professionalism should be borne in mind when considering the experiences of nurses and learners at work.

Whether nurses are 'professionals' or not is unaffected by the notion of the 'good nurse'. However, the idea of the good nurse needs to be addressed by those who are involved in nursing. What is the relationship, for example, of the good nurse to the doctor? Should the good nurse be obedient or questioning? What role ought the good nurse to play in relation to trade unions or professional bodies? What should the good nurse do in response to attacks on the NHS? Should the good nurse be politically deaf, dumb and blind?

From these questions, it becomes apparent that the notion of the 'good nurse' comes with a set of implicit prescriptions. First and foremost the idea strongly reflects Nightingale's emphasis on character rather than skills. The idea of the good nurse does not make reference to a highly skilled, specialized or professional worker. To be a good nurse seems to rest on personal attributes: kindness, patience, compassion, and understanding. Nurses are, in the usual words, born not made.

The idea also reflects the belief that women should be silent, passive, and apolitical. While men may decide to wage war and to fight in wars, it is the women who will quietly, without judgement, tend to the wounds which men inflict upon each other. (The idea of the 'good nurse' seldom appears to encompass the belief that men can also be carers.) At the same time, the good nurse should not be shouting out about what she sees, but should silently and with acquiescence clear up the mess left by others.

The potential dangers, of a pursuit of professionalization and equality with others, to those who do not wish to hear from these silent carers become apparent. These 'silent carers' do have a voice, which is occasionally used and is normally attended to. It is not necessary to embark on the 'closure' of the occupation by professionalizing it and the exclusion of the unqualified in order to speak out. It is up to nurses themselves to decide how they think a 'good nurse' should behave.

However, there are many changes both proposed and underway which will affect nurses and nursing. It is to these that the next chapter will be addressed.

Notes

1 For an appreciation of some of the different perspectives on nurses see Kiger, A.M. (1985) '"Mirror, mirror on the wall . . ." Some reflections on the image' *in* Proceedings of the 19th Annual Study Day of the Nursing Studies Association, *The Politics of Power*, University of Edinburgh, The Nursing Studies Association.

2 The way in which nurses are portrayed in the electronic media is reported by Kalisch and Kalisch (1986).

3 These findings are broadly similar to those reported by Kiger (1985) *in* University of Edinburgh, p. 7.

4 See Kiger (1985) *in* University of Edinburgh, p. 7.

5 Ehrenreich and English (1973) p. 36; see also Salvage on this point (1985), pp. 18ff.

6 See also Logan who points out that paramedical groups are specializing in areas which used to be the domain of nurses (1986) 'The Scottish Experience (*Project 2000*)' *Nursing Times*, 27 August, 82:35, p. 49.

7 Young (1983), p. 82.

8 Oakley, A. (1984) 'The importance of being a nurse' *Nursing Times*, 12 December 80:50, p. 26.

9 Some would strongly dispute the traditional view of nursing as being women's work – see Kiger *in* University of Edinburgh (1985), p. 4.

10 Carpenter (1978) *in* Dingwall and McIntosh (eds), p. 99.

11 Batchelor (1984) *in* Duncan and McLachlan (eds), p. 73.

12 Salvage (1985), p. 92.

11

Change and More Change

The National Health Service is in the throes of many changes which will dramatically affect the nurses' experience of their work. Changes in management emphasis and style appear to be producing divisions between management and carers. The government initiatives to increase the amount of private health care find some echo among the ranks of nurses. Quite a number of nurses could be persuaded to work in the private sector. The changes being implemented as a result of *Project 2000* are by no means universally approved of by nurses. In particular there is resistance to the phasing out of the enrolled nurse grade. Divisions within the ranks of women who care for patients seem likely. The present 'closed system' of nurse training will go with the movement of nurse training to polytechnics and colleges. However, the anti-academic sentiments in nursing may produce difficulties when the new nurses enter the system. The move towards greater care in the community will substantially affect the lives of women: as carers who are paid and those who are unpaid. The 'low-cost solution' to the rising costs of health care may end up being paid for by women.

A number of far-reaching changes are presently being recommended or implemented within the NHS. These changes will substantially affect nurses and nursing. The changes focus variously on the increasing promotion of private health-care provision; the privatization of various aspects of the NHS; changes in the style and organization of management in Health Authorities; a change in emphasis towards preventative care and care in the community, with a reduced reliance on hospital-based care; and, finally changes in nurse education.

The move towards increasing privatization of health-care provision means that nurses will have greater choice as to where they work. I asked the leavers whether they would work, or if they had ever worked, in the private health-care sector. Only a small proportion of the leavers had worked at some time in the private sector. Under half of the leavers would consider working in the private sector, often with reservations:

> Yes, I would work in the private sector. I think the private sector is probably better in a lot of ways than the National Health hospitals, and eventually we will all be private anyway . . . It will be a bad thing for a lot of people, especially the unemployed and the elderly, it will be a terrible thing, but you can see it happening. (Enrolled Nurse)

Quite a few nurses had considered and rejected the idea of working in private sector. The rest were adamant that they would not consider working in private health care.

> No, DEFINITELY NOT. I disagree with it. I mean it's your decision if you want to have private care, then fine but I don't see why the NHS should pay for your training and then using beds in the NHS – I think it's unethical – and using laboratories. No, definitely not. (Sister)

Some nurses, but they were a minority, were obviously staunch defenders of the NHS. More pragmatic reasons were given by many of the nurses who had rejected working in the private sector:

> I prefer to keep safe and secure in the NHS. (Enrolled Nurse)

> I've nothing against private medicine – I think perhaps it may be a bit slow for me. (Sister)

Overall, just over half of the leavers would consider working in the private sector.[1] The issue was very topical at the time. A private hospital locally was nearing completion and a number of nurses in particular specialties had been approached. Only one of the leavers interviewed was actually going to work in the private sector.

The relationship between nurse and patient changes in the private sector. The patient is paying directly for every aspect of the care which is given. The nurse, in other words, is being paid directly and obviously for the service given. The nurse becomes more like a servant. Patients may feel they are paying for every smile and every attention they get. And as Chapman points out: '. . . where payment for services is overt, as in the case of private nursing, many nurses express their dislike of the situation seeing themselves relegated to the role of a servant'.[2] Private patients may be more demanding and less grateful than NHS patients. Thus, a district nurse reported that: 'They expected everything there and then'. It is more difficult to maintain a self-image of being the sort of person who wants to help and care when you are faced with patients who demand what you prefer to offer freely. The patient may not be judged by the nurse but the nurse comes to be judged by the patient. The notion of 'service' is harder to maintain in an environment in which everything is obviously paid for.

The privatization of health care is also taking place through hiving off parts of the NHS to private contractors. To date this form of privatization has tended to focus on cleaning, catering, laundry, etc. There are, however, plans to extend this privatization to other aspects such as pathology laboratories, etc. I did not ask specifically about this aspect of privatization but a few nurses did comment on it. There were concerns that standards might fall if private contractors were to take over. There were also concerns about the 'special relationships' with staff which would be affected by privatization.

> . . . if they bring the private people in, I don't know how things are going to be cleaned. I mean the ladies that we have, we have a lovely relationship with them as well and if you ask them to clean a certain item you know that it is going to be done properly . . . It's gone out to tender and the tender has been accepted . . . Now are they going to expect the nurses in the future to do some of the cleaning, the qualified nurses? (Sister)

This latter concern of nurses, that the competitive tendering would reduce the numbers of ancillary workers to the extent that nurses might be forced to carry out their work, has been voiced also by the RCN.[3] The potential problems caused by privatization were also tied up with efficiency seeking measures which often involved reducing the numbers of ancillary staff.

> We haven't got our own porter now. And some [porters] are a wee bit reluctant to come in here and we have to watch everything that is done to make sure that it is done – you have got to stand over them – it makes our job harder. (Sister)

The need to 'stand over' ancillary workers who are either not attached to a specific unit or who are employed by private contractors adds to the concerns of nurses. Not only do they have to think about their own work, they have to be constantly checking and re-checking the work of others. Instead of having a trusting relationship with ancillary staff, there may develop a division between NHS and non-NHS employees. As Cousins remarks, with contracting out 'ancillary workers are no longer part of the health-care team, but become isolated and separated by the factory-like regime of work which conflicts with the patient care values and priorities of other health care workers'.[4]

The moves to greater privatization in health care have been accompanied by a change of approach towards management in the NHS. Following the recommendations of the Griffiths report, the notion of 'general managers' has been introduced from the private, commercial sector into the NHS. Changes in the style and organization of management have taken place. A move away from the 'labyrinthine' process of consultation[5] which was 'consensus management' has taken place towards a system of general management where decision making can be speeded up and made more dynamic. At the same time, managerial responsibility is meant to be pushed as far down the management line as possible.[6] Perhaps most crucially of all, the introduction of general management was accompanied by an increasing emphasis on efficiency and value for money.[7] As part of this, performance indicators (PIs) are monitored. By counting the number of patients who are admitted and discharged; the bed-occupancy rate; the number of day-patients; the number of calls made by a district nurse, etc. it is believed that an indication of the performance of various health-care workers and of the service can be obtained. The PI does give information which enables comparisons to be made regarding the throughput of, say, orthopaedic consultants in different parts of the Health Authority. It does have some use as a management tool in helping identify poorly performing units, and individuals. However, PIs leave out of account the quality of service that is provided. For example, no account is taken of the number of patients who are re-admitted having been discharged from hospital too quickly. This is, it should be noted, technically feasible, but not carried out. PIs do not measure patient satisfaction or the morale of the workforce. It is a 'narrow engineering model of health care'[8] which 'tends to under-rate the experience of being treated'.[9] Although PIs may be useful they may also be a dangerous tool to use if their limitations are not remembered. When the general manager's contract is examined it is found to be a short-term contract with special payment for savings which have been made in the service. A sense of survival may ensure that general managers pay greater attention to the immediate and obvious results of PIs than to the hidden costs of a qualitatively poorer service. The 'new managerialism' introduces tensions between management and carers.[10]

Of course, as Cousins points out, the managers themselves are in a 'professional strangehold': 'if the new managers are successful in running an underfunded service and making further cuts, the government will continue to reduce the Health Service budget'.[11]

General managers were being brought into the Health Authority as the interviews were being conducted. It was too early to ask any questions which related to the effects of the introduction of these managers. I did, however, ask nurses opinions of the management at district headquarters. And, as noted in Chapter 8, opinions of management were not high. As time went by, the introduction of non-nurses into management was being commented on more often by those I spoke to. There was a general feeling that 'nurses should be in charge of nurses'. At the same time, experience of working in the NHS – at some level – was felt to be necessary.

> I think they perhaps should come and try and get a more real life grasp of what it's like on the ward. I don't think anybody who hasn't done nursing can have a real life grasp really. I'm sure they can't. (Staff Nurse)

The fact that a number of general managers had come from the retail trade was often mentioned, parallels being made between patients and tins of baked beans or other groceries:

> One of the administrators was saying he was so impressed by the way was it Sainsbury's was run, no it was Marks & Spencers – it was just like saying the patient on your left-hand side is a bag of Marks & Spencers' cheese and onion crisps – we're going to get it working as well . . . (Staff Nurse)

The different ethos of the general managers was also identified:

> I think it permeates through the district – the elderly people are not a high priority. Their interest is being abandoned to balance the books. (Charge Nurse)

General managers from outside the Health Service were also seen as wanting to have the same status symbols of expensively decorated offices and luxurious furnishings as they were perceived to have had elsewhere.

> They had that place [HQ] upgraded. The money they spent on that when they are supposed to be short of money in the Health Service was obscene. They had fitted carpets, they had all this decorating done, they had ornate pieces on the ceiling picked out in gold paint and new desks and they sit there in their luxurious central heating and tell us that we've to switch the heating off . . . and the trouble we had to go through to get it back on . . . (Sister)

Just as the implementation of the Salmon recommendations resulted in a growth of trade unionism,[12] so the introduction of general managers is seen as widening the gap between workers and management. It may result in a more militant workforce. Some nurses see the growing gap happening everywhere in Britain. Others feel that no one is now looking after their interests: 'these general managers just seem to have come in and taken over, nobody seems to be representing us' (Sister). Royal Commissions may comment on the need not to abuse the goodwill of those who work in the Health Service.[13] However, the introduction of general managers with different aims and priorities is unlikely to increase morale in the NHS or, as Griffiths envisaged 'to capitalise on the existing high levels of dedication and expertise'.[14] It is evident that managers have been paying rather more attention to some parts of the Griffiths recommendations than others. For example, 'optimum manpower levels'[15] appear to have received greater attention than management training and career development – at least amongst nurses.

Another change which is being effected is the move to greater emphasis on care in the community with a corresponding move away from the present domination of hospital-based care.[16] Many criticisms have been made of the way the move to community care is being effected. It has, for instance, been seen as a 'low-cost solution' in which the burden of care falls on family, friends and neighbours.[17]

The changes to 'community care' operate in two main areas. Firstly, patients from psychiatric hospitals are being 'rehabilitated' so that they can return to the community they came from. This movement has caused quite a few problems. Some long-stay patients have no relatives or contacts at all with the place they originally came from. For many long-stay patients the town they came from has changed out of all recognition in the last 20 or 30 years. Patients who have been in a psychiatric hospital for decades see it as their home and the nurses have become their friends. Moving such patients out of their homes is a traumatic experience. From a sheltered environment they move into a community which often shuns and ridicules the ex-mental-patient. Accustomed to fixed routines and a fairly predictable environment such patients are likely to feel 'lost' outside the hospital. Many nurses are concerned about their patients' moves into the community.

It's not fair on them. Some of them have got no idea. They will be conned by a lot of people, because they don't even have the idea of money or the value of money, and they are so trusting, they trust everyone with their money and they expect everyone to do the same. They are going too fast with it – if they had proper places, safe places – but they've not that, have they? (Pupil)

Appraisal interviews to gauge the suitability of patients for moving out of hospital were being conducted at the same time as our research. Some nurses were indignant at the whole process:

> We have had resettlement teams coming round interviewing the patients and to me it's like, how can I put it, it's like a cattle market. They are coming to see *our* patients – if they are a good patient, and they are not incontinent, who doesn't need a maximum amount of care, they will take them. If they are a management problem or doubly incontinent they don't want to know. The patient is brought in, doesn't know what on earth is going on. He could have been in here 40 or 50 years and if he's a good patient then they say yes, we will accept him when the hospital closes. And this is their home – this is all they know . . . (Enrolled Nurse)

There is a symbiotic relationship between nurses and patients in the areas of mental illness and mental handicap in particular. The relationships are often based on friendship rather than on duty. Long-standing relationships are built up. And patients are not alone in having to face the move 'into the community'. For the pyschiatric nurses who themselves may have spent decades in the hospital, a similar move into the community has to be made. Because mental hospitals are often in rural areas where there is little alternative employment, nurses may also have to move out of the area. If psychiatric nurses wish to pursue nursing in the community they have to undergo further training. The resources for this training are not always immediately available. It would not be surprising if many psychiatric nurses, with their expensive training, were to leave nursing altogether. Yet there is no predicted downturn in the level of mental illness or mental disturbance. Indeed, it has been shown that high levels of unemployment, as tolerated at the moment, result in a greater incidence of mental as well as physical ill health.[18] The skills of psychiatric nurses will continue to be needed. Yet will there be a place for them to work? Many psychiatric nurses feel their future to be insecure. Their employment prospects are unclear. Not surprisingly, morale amongst psychiatric nurses is not high. (There is some evidence from the leavers interviewed that the movement from psychiatric hospital to community is proceeding apace. Six of the mental illness nurse leavers were taking up posts in the community, although not always as nurses. Three were continuing to work as nurses, two were moving into the social service side and another to a charitable association.)

Another move towards greater care in the community is the attempt to increasingly care for patients in their own homes and minimize their length of stay in hospital. Patients who are recovering from surgery are returned to their own homes much more speedily than a few years ago. There is no doubt that patients are often very keen to return home. Sometimes, however, patients are sent home too soon.

> They send people out sometimes too early; they send them out with obvious infections that they haven't done anything about. It's more or less when you walk in, you say 'I'll get the doctor to see you straight away'. They sometimes send them out – they haven't lately because we now have the liaison which do try and not do it – but they have come out to me on a Friday afternoon with no back-up at all. That's been horrendous. (District Nurse)

> [In midwifery] It is routine to discharge somebody on their fifth day, whether or not . . . without somebody looking at the family unit as a whole and I, for example, have made recommendations, on very, very few occasions, where I feel they need some more supervision or there is a housing problem, and found that they've still been discharged on their fifth day. And that happens not just in midwifery . . . (Sister)

At the same time, there is a growing demand for geriatric beds in hospitals which cannot be met. As a result, increasing numbers of elderly people will have to be cared for outside the NHS. Many elderly people will go into private nursing homes – another aspect of government policy designed to increase the privatization of health care. Indeed, without a large private sector, many elderly people could not have been moved out of hospital.

> There are so many of these nursing homes about now. If all those ladies and gentlemen were out 'on the district', we wouldn't know what to do. (District Nurse)

(It should be noted that although private homes may give '24-hour care', district nurses may still have to go and do dressings, insulin injections, etc.) However, for those patients who do not enter private nursing homes, the burden of caring for them often falls on the community nursing service and on patients' families.

The burden of caring within families normally falls most heavily on women. The policy of increasing 'care in the community' may make it even more difficult for women to undertake paid employment.[19] At a time when the value of 'family life' is being stressed by those on the political Right, this policy will ensure that even greater pressure is exerted on women to stay at home. (One result of this, similar to the post World War programmes, will be to 'keep the jobs for the men'. In turn this may mean that unemployment can be reduced to 'reasonable' levels by social rather than economic policies.) Research suggests, however, that family life actually suffers when caring is undertaken at home.[20] Women who are carers often feel that their children or husbands receive inadequate attention when they have an older relative to care for.[21]

At the moment, health care in the UK is still very much hospital orientated. This orientation to hospital-based health care and hospital-based nurse training is frequently bemoaned.[22] There may be, as one health visitor suggested, a tendency for hospital-based nurses not to appreciate the realities facing patients outside hospital:

> Whereas all nurses on the community have spent quite a few years in hospitals, if only for the training, they have a good insight into hospital life. The reverse isn't so. And some hospital nurses have very little community experience . . . I think it's all too easy for them if they see just a child in hospital with parents visiting, without appreciating the wider aspects of a child at home, where the mother will not necessarily be . . . motivated. (Health Visitor)

The planned increase in attention to nursing in the community will obviously help maximize the benefits which are to be found both in hospital and in community care.

Community medicine, although growing, is still in its infancy and having its teething troubles.[23] Community nursing services are currently being increased. However, it appears, according to the nurses I spoke to, that this increase is not keeping up with demand:

> It sounds a good idea but there are not the resources to cope with it. I think it's going to be a disaster unless they really get a lot more staff and have a lot more resources to deal with it. The idea is a nice one, it's always far nicer for people to be in small units and at home but they really still need a lot of care and very often they need someone there monitoring them. I can't see that it can work as things stand at the moment. There simply isn't enough staff. (District Nurse)

From those working in the community there is broad agreement that the move to greater care within the community is a good one, provided the necessary resources and back-up are available.

It could be super if it's done properly and the money is there.
District nurses cannot do baths any longer, it is very sad. Patients
just have to give themselves a good wash down if they can.
(Health Visitor)

In the longer term many more nurses will be required to work in the
community. It has previously been pointed out that there is scope for a
greater role for health visitors and district nurses in the community.[24]
Even if local authorities are given responsibility for care in the
community,[25] there will continue to be an increasing demand for the
services of nurses. Firstly, in caring for patients who have recently
received hospital treatment and, secondly as a result of the intended
increase in preventative health care. In nurse training the emphasis is
still very much towards hospital nursing. However, many nurses
were keen to move into 'the community' (see also Appendix 10). A
major barrier to that movement is seen to be the restricted number of
places on training courses and the shortage of permanent jobs in
community nursing. One health visitor on completing her training
found there was no post for her in the health authority:

Really we have heard so much about community care. This was
one of the reasons I decided to do health visiting because I could
foresee such a great need for it. But it's all talk and there seems to
be little money going into that area. (Health Visitor)

Perhaps the most far reaching changes of all for nurses, will result
from the recommendations from the UKCC in *Project 2000*. The
function of the United Kingdom Central Council for Nursing, Midwifery and Health Visiting is 'to establish and improve standards of
training and professional conduct for nurses, midwives and health
visitors'.[26] Their report was concerned to 'carry out a wide-ranging
review of educational preparation' for these groups of 'nurses'.[27] The
recommendations of the UKCC (which were agreed to by the Social
Services Secretary in May, 1988) will mean fundamental changes in
the system of nurse training and in the structure of nursing itself. The
recommendations are wide-ranging: (1) the abolition of the grade of
enrolled nurse. In future there will only be one gate of entry for
nurses. A single grade of nurse a 'knowledgeable doer' 'will embrace
much of the work of the present two levels of nurse'.[28] Also envisaged
is a more advanced grade of specialist practitioner, as well as a support
worker: 'the helper'. (2) nurse training will be transferred from Schools
of Nursing to polytechnics. A common foundation programme of up
to 2 years for all nurses will be followed by a 'branch' programme[29] for
particular specialities. (3) nurse learners will be 'supernumerary' on
the wards. This means that learners' contribution to 'service' will be
reduced from 60 per cent to 20 per cent.

The repercussions of these changes can only be guessed at until they come into effect. Although the amount and accuracy of information which the nurses and learners had obtained about *Project 2000* was variable, quite a degree of scepticism about the plans was expressed. Discussion focused on three main aspects. The first, and least popular is the intention to phase out the grade of enrolled nurses.

> If you just make it staff nurses and auxiliaries, there's going to be a missing link between them. I mean, SENs are qualified nurses and they can give the care and leave the staff nurses to get on with the office side of it and running the ward. No, I don't think they should get rid of them. (Student)

Will the slightly trained 'helper' who, it is envisaged by the UKCC, may only be trained for 3 months[30] be taking over some of the enrolled nurse's work?

> It seems funny, doesn't it? If they scrap ENs, they are going to have to give nursing assistants extra training so that they can do basic nursing duties. (Enrolled Nurse)

If the duties of the enrolled nurse are taken up by the 'knowledgeable doer', what will it involve? Although there are plans to develop 'specialist practitioners' who will be highly trained and skilled nurses, a deskilling lower down in the ranks of the registered nurse may occur.

> It will end up the same kind of system but without the different actual grading, you are going to get the senior staff nurses and junior staff nurses and just going to be doing what the enrolled nurses were doing, and getting the same responsibility as ENs get now. (Mary)

In any case, will staff nurses be prepared to spend a great deal of their time on bedside nursing? Will they accept what must be seen as a downgrading in responsibility? Will there be a great deal of squabbling and animosity as to who is to be in the office?

> I can't see the staff nurses actually preferring to rush round on the wards doing all the nasty horrible jobs when they can sit in the office doing sort of nice jobs. (Ann)

There was an implicit acceptance that many staff nurses did not want to be on the wards. Staff nurses were seen, especially by the learners, as wanting to move away, as soon as possible, from ward work towards the office and promotion. The potential competition between staff nurses to be 'in the office' was a recurring theme.

I think when they do get rid of enrolled nurses a lot of the staff nurses are going to have a shock because they are going to have to spend a lot more time with patients . . . I think that's why they go in for their SRN some of them because they know they've only got to be with the patients for 3 years and then after that they can work up to Sister. (Clare)

Enrolled nurses are felt by many nurses to have a particular contribution to make:

. . . we need more down-to-earth nurses who seem to have a lot of common sense and can talk to patients, and you find this very strongly with enrolled nurses and say, cleaners, they seem to be able to get on a lot better with the ordinary type of person, the ordinary working-class person. (Staff Nurse)

At senior nurse level there is also little enthusiasm for the phasing out of the enrolled nurse grade. Enrolled nurses are variously seen to be the 'backbone of the psychiatric services'; 'excellent bedside nurses' who give the 'real basic bedside care'. It has been observed that 'there must be people who are excellent nurses in their own particular sphere who have neither the ambition nor the capacity to become the fully rounded nurse envisaged in the Report'.[31] Enrolled nurses may not want to convert. They have a great deal of patient contact. This contact might well be lost if they become registered nurses. 'I think the higher up you go the further away from patients you are going . . . it is the lower grades who spend more time with the patients' (Patricia). Some nurses felt enrolled nurses had few, if any, career aspirations and they were quite happy with their lot (a view not always shared by enrolled nurses themselves – see Chapter 6).

. . . enrolled nurses are there purely to work with the patients, they've not got any career ideas you know. They've got what they wanted and that's all they want. (Julie)

On the other hand, many nurses feel that enrolled nurses presently get a raw deal:

I'm inclined to think that they are regarded as second-class nurses. And yet they are very caring girls and many make excellent nurses. No, I think perhaps it will be a mistake to get rid of them on the whole but, on the other hand, I think in a lot of places they are just a glorified auxiliary. (Sister)

The responsibilities which enrolled nurses have been given in the past are already being whittled away. For example, enrolled nurses mentioned that they used to be left in charge of wards but that happens much less often now. Enrolled nurses also used to be able to check drugs and they are no longer allowed to do so. In this Health Authority, at least, steps appear to being taken to clear the way for the implementation of the UKCC's recommendations.

There has been a tendency within nursing to mis-use enrolled nurses. There has been an acceptance that enrolled nurses do not wish to have careers and few attempts appear made to develop systematically the skills of enrolled nurses. Partly this is due to the feeling that there are 'too many chiefs and not enough Indians' within the ranks of nurses. Enrolled nurses make good 'Indians' who will stay in their place. For a variety of reasons, there appears to have been a substantial waste of enrolled nurses' talent and potential.

There are other, practical, drawbacks in removing the grade of enrolled nurse, such as problems of recruitment and finding additional nurses to cover for the enrolled nurses who choose to do conversion courses.

> Where is all this extra workforce going to come from and all this extra money? Because they are going to have to re-train all the enrolled nurses who want to be re-trained. So I don't see how it's all going to come off. (Katy)

> I mean they're having trouble recruiting people anyway. It's going to be worse if they make it [the entrance qualifications] even higher. It's not as if it's a job which is really highly paid and everyone wants to go in it, is it? (Sally)

If there are too few potential recruits, will it mean that more and more unqualified staff will have to be used? It may mean that recommendations regarding ratios of qualified to unqualified staff will increasingly have to be disregarded.

Will the enrolled nurse of today become the 'helper' of tomorrow? 'it seems a shame for those that would make very good nurses but haven't got the qualifications – it doesn't seem fair on them' (Wendy). Already about half of the nursing workforce are unqualified.[32] Will it mean that there will be fewer nurses (and fewer women) who are qualified?[33] Can the much reduced amount of training mean an even lower salary for the helper compared to the enrolled nurse? Is it simply a means by which cheaper care can be given to NHS patients? Does it mean a real division between the ranks and the officers in nursing?

There were many issues raised about the practicalities of enrolled nurses 'converting' to the Register. From both student and staff nurses, there were worries that enrolled nurses would be allowed to register without having had to obtain the same level of qualifications.

For enrolled nurses, difficulties associated with taking a conversion course were outlined:

> having qualified 15 years ago, I would have to revert back to student-nurse plus taking a considerable pay cut – as most of us have not got the academic qualifications required: it would make it virtually impossible for us. A crash course and exams would be a much fairer and sensible way of upgrading SENs who have been qualified *x* number of years. (Senior Enrolled Nurse)

> . . . what happens if I leave to have a family? What chance have I got of getting a job back after 5 years. My only hope is to leave nursing if the present situation continues. (Enrolled Nurse)

Many enrolled nurses voiced fears about their job prospects, despite many assurances to the contrary. Rumours abounded regarding the scarcity of conversion courses and the number of O levels required from enrolled nurses who wished to convert. It is perhaps a measure of the distrust of management (and of the government) amongst nurses that such a large degree of uncertainty, fear and worry about their job security continues to exist. It was obvious that many enrolled nurses lacked confidence in their ability to undertake further studying.

Project 2000 recommends that nurse training should take place in polytechnics rather than in Schools of Nursing. This means that nurse learners will not be isolated from other disciplines. Only a small proportion of nurses felt training nurses in polytechnics would be a good idea.

> I think it's a wonderful idea because you have such a narrow view of the world. I mean I've been in uniform since I was 17 if you think about it and I have got a very narrow view of what's outside. And nursing isn't just about looking after sick people, it's also about people who can become sick. Perhaps I wouldn't get as many admissions if there was somebody out there looking after them. (Sister)

This comment makes clear the present emphasis in nurse training on ward experience, on practical experience. Of course, as the RCN points out 'nursing can only be taught and learnt in the context of giving care'.[34] However, the other side of health care, the preventative, community-based model is relatively neglected at the moment.[35] The benefits of a college-based rather than NHS-based training would be obvious if a broader and longer-term view of health care were to be pursued there as envisaged in *Project 2000*.[36] Other benefits in being trained in polytechnics and colleges were mentioned. For example, nursing officers referred to the benefits of 'keeping up' with other professionals and that Schools of Nursing 'don't do the image of nursing any good'.

Criticisms about moving out of Schools of Nursing were also made.

> [In midwifery] if something is going on in the delivery suite, we will phone the School and say 'look there's something special going on, do you want to send a couple of students up to see?' It's a different set-up than in a general school [of nursing].

A nursing officer made explicit one fear about nurse learners moving into the sphere of higher education: the potential threat to the 'good order' of nursing.

> To be honest with you I think there are a lot of left-wing elements – stuff that's talked in corridors today. Hopefully they will be mature enough to absorb it, sort it out and chew it round and spit it out and come out wiser for it. I wouldn't like to see that element brought into the profession from these colleges. In as much as well 'we strike or . . .' I could see more conflict in nursing . . .

The advantages of the 'closed system' of Schools of Nursing in minimizing conflict and reducing the input of 'different' ideas are obvious. Similarly, a Sister pointed out that nurses trained in colleges would not be loyal to a particular hospital, they would be professionals first and NHS nurses second.

However, the main criticism of basing training in colleges and away from Schools of Nursing focused on the greater emphasis given to studying and a corresponding reduction in the amount of time spent on the clinical side. The 'contribution to service' by nurse learners would be reduced from 60 per cent to 20 per cent. Learners would be supernumerary on the wards. That is, learners would not be counted in when staffing complements were being arranged. The position of learners on the wards under the recommendations of *Project 2000* is not very clear. Will it mean as suggested in the *Hospital and Health Services Review* editorial: 'Watch dear, but don't get in the way'? or: 'Thank goodness the students are coming next week and we can catch up on all those jobs'?[37]

Most of the nurses I talked to really liked the idea that learners were to be supernumerary. For example, a final year student nurse felt it was a good idea if learners could: ' . . . go out to a ward 1 or 2 days a week, as an observer and put your skills that you are learning gradually into play'. Some of the learners and the qualified nurses resented the fact that students and pupils were often treated as simply a pair of hands. Learners were sometimes felt to be used as 'fodder' to keep the wards going in the absence of sufficient qualified staff.

Most nurses, however, did not like the implied move in *Project 2000* towards greater emphasis on theoretical input to nurse training. There were many, many comments about the need for practical rather than academic skills in nursing. A dislike of the 'academic' was often mentioned.

> . . . in psychiatric the more experience you get on the wards the better because the whole thing is about dealing with people really. I think the sooner they get out onto the wards working with the patients the better. I don't think it helps coming into a job like this with a head full of theory. (Enrolled Nurse)

> Half the thing with nursing is that you cannot teach a person how, not [how to] behave, but you go onto a ward and its a confidence building I think, from day one – and its the rapport you have with your patient. And you gradually become more confident. (Sister)

As mentioned earlier, this belief, whatever its accuracies, very neatly ensures that many nurses do not aspire to become more knowledgeable academically or theoretically. Thus, nurses stay in their place. Such a belief is perpetuated, of course, by being passed on to learners with the bundle of ideas they receive as they go through their training.

> Maybe that would produce better results when it came to the exams, but once you've qualified, nursing is about being with people, not sitting at desks writing, isn't it? . . . I mean anybody can be brilliant mentally but it's how you are dealing with the people themselves that makes you a nurse, not what you've got up here, you know. (Yvonne)

Similarities between 'degree nurses' and the proposals of *Project 2000* to base nurse training more firmly in the higher education sector were sometimes drawn. No positive comments were made in this respect.

> It's a bit like the degree they did a few years ago. I remember when I was training, degree nurses coming into hospital – I think I resented them. Because nursing is just practice and it's not all theory. I think they're tending to make nurses too technical and the nursing as I was trained to do it, has been taken away from you. (Staff Nurse)

Just as there was resistance to the idea of a greater academic input into nurse training, many learners did not like the idea of spending a greater amount of time studying. There were differences in this respect between the students and pupils.

While nearly half of the students said that they felt spending more time in school was a good idea, only one pupil felt the same way. On the other hand, nearly half the pupils and only one student said they became bored or fell asleep when in school.

> My tutor will tell you that I often doze off. I don't actually fall asleep but I find it very difficult to sit at a desk . . . my eyes just go. And I'm not tired, it's just with sitting in the same position all day. (Barbara)

There does seem to be a division between the students and pupils where the former are keener to gain greater theoretical knowledge.

Nearly half of the students and pupils suggested it would be better to have shorter but more frequent spells in school, consolidating what they had learned during each allocation. Currently, learners move from one allocation to a second one before returning to the school for 'consolidation'. The delay in being able to discuss experiences and what had been learned with peers and tutors was clearly regretted. This was especially the case with regard to negative experiences which had occurred to one or two pupils and which they wanted to report.

For some learners a reduction in the percentage of time spent in practical work means that some of the pressure they felt in school to 'cram things in' would be relieved. The need for sufficient theoretical input was also voiced: 'Friends say nursing is about being on the wards. Well it is, but you are no use on the ward if you don't know what you are doing really' (Julie). A greater length of time spent on theory could also, if learners were really to be supernumerary, enhance the quality of the experience which learners had on the wards.

Tied in with the idea of a college-based training is the pursuit of professionalization (see Chapter 10). As accredited professionals nurses could hope to be given greater respect and status within the health care team. Similarly they would be in a better position to secure substantial increases in salary. They would have a greater chance of affecting the way health care is delivered, e.g. whether health care should increasingly be focused on preventative rather than on the curative model. However, getting rid of the enrolled nurse grade, with its lower entrance qualifications, is part of the move towards professionalization. Robinson, for example, argues that in *Project*

2000 'the professionalising sector of nursing won the day and reneged on its less powerful practitioner colleagues'.[38]

At the moment, nursing can be seen as being 'diluted' by the presence of enrolled nurses with relatively few academic qualifications. After all, how can nurses aspire to professional status when many of their colleagues wish to remain at ward level and closely concerned with patient care (and the stereotyped women's work)? Nurses who do not wish to 'rise from the ranks' and challenge the authority of other health care professionals, will be of little help in pursuing the status of professional. By this line of argument, nursing will continue to be (merely?) a semi-profession.[39]

The debates surrounding *Project 2000* have not been fully explored here and they certainly cannot be resolved here.[40] However, the very real fears which have been expressed by many of these nurses will have to be taken into account when the recommendations of *Project 2000* are implemented.

The changes outlined above are far-reaching changes which will have a fundamental impact on the NHS. The trouble is that more changes are needed if the status and working conditions of nurses and their patients are to be improved. Changes are needed to increase the opportunities for women to combine nursing with domestic responsibilities; to realize their own potential and career aspirations; and most importantly, to be able to do the job they want to do to their own satisfaction.

The changes being effected in the NHS at the moment are exceedingly broad in focus. They are structural changes affecting all those involved in health care. They are changes which have, in the main, resulted from political ideologies; (it has, after all, been a political decision rather than a popular one to limit the amount of resources we devote to the NHS. Resistance to spending more money on the Health Service comes from within the ranks of government not from the electorate) the assumed benefits of competition; the assumed superiority of management methods in the private sector; the assumed benefits of 'self-care' rather than collective social responsibility.[41,42] The move to greater care in the community may have been favoured because it could involve cost savings. Whatever the reason, the potential benefits of being cared for at home rather than in hospital cannot be gainsaid. The changes envisaged by the UKCC in *Project 2000* may have been pursued with the interests of the 'professionals' at heart. But it seems likely that they could also act as the cornerstone for a fundamental re-orientation of the provision of health care.

Notes

1 It would be surprising if more nurses were antagonistic to private health care given the example set by many consultants who are only too happy to take on private patients.
2 Chapman (1979) *in* Colledge and Jones, pp. 122–3.
3 RCN (1986) *in* DHSS, p. 25.
4 Cousins (1987), p. 178.
5 Griffiths (1983), p. 14.
6 Griffiths (1983), p. 2.
7 For an analysis of the 'new managerialism' see Carpenter (1978) *in* Dingwall and McIntosh, and Cousins (1987), Chapter 2.
8 Davidson (1987), p. 48.
9 Davidson (1987), p. 5.
10 Cousins (1987), p. 171.
11 Cousins (1987), p. 165.
12 See Carpenter (1978) *in* Dingwall and McIntosh.
13 Merrison (1979), p. 166.
14 Griffiths (1983), p. 13.
15 Griffiths (1983), p. 7.
16 See Draper, P. *et al. in* Tuckett (ed.) (1976), p. 283.
17 Cousins (1987) p. 157.
18 See Whitehead (1987), pp. 19–22.
19 It is pointed out in Cousins (1987), p. 158, citing Finch, that this will act so as to increase the sexual division of labour by depending on 'the substantial and consistent input of women's unpaid labour in the home, whilst at the same time effectively excluding them from the labour market and increasing their economic and personal dependence on men' (Finch 1984, p. 6).
20 See Ungerson, C. (1987) *Policy is Personal*, London, Tavistock, p. 129.
21 For some moving accounts of the repercussions of 'care in the community' see Ungerson ibid.
22 See, for example, RCN (1986); Salvage (1985).
23 See, for example, Cumberlege (1986).
24 Merrison (1979), p. 79.
25 See the recommendations of Griffiths, E.R. (1988) *Community Care: Agenda for Action*, A Report to the Secretary of State for Social Services, London, HMSO.
26 UKCC (1986), p. 3.
27 UKCC (1986), p. 3.
28 UKCC (1987) *Project 2000: the Final Proposals*, Project Paper 9, London, UKCC. February, p. 5.
29 ibid. p. 6.
30 UKCC (1986) para. 5.37, p. 43.
31 *Hospital and Health Services Review* (1986) (editorial), *Hospital and Health Services Review*, September, 82, 5, p. 194.
32 See Merrison (1979), p. 195.
33 As COHSE suggest, see UKCC (1986), p. 39.
34 RCN quoted *in* Merrison (1979), p. 202.

35 WHO (1974), p. 12.
36 UKCC (1986), p. 33.
37 *Hospital and Health Services Review* (1986), p. 194.
38 Robinson, J. (1986) 'Through the minefield – and into the sun?' *Senior Nurse*, 4:6, p. 8; see also Salvage (1985), p. 86.
39 For an analysis of nursing and other 'semi-professions', see Etzioni (ed.) (1969).
40 For a wider appreciation of the debates see Martin, L. (1986) 'Future tense', *Nursing Times*, 13 August, pp. 48–9; Robinson (1986) *Nursing Times* (1987) 'Ready for lift-off' (editorial), *Nursing Times*, 28 January, 83, 4, pp. 16–19; Devlin B. (1987) 'An unreal brave new world?', *Nursing Times*, 6 May, 83:18, pp. 29–30; Dickson, N. (1986) 'The future with confidence', *Nursing Times*, 5 November, 82:45, pp. 50–1, and, of course, the recommendations of the UKCC (1986).
41 Salvage (1985), p. 152.
42 Of course, it needs to be remembered that health care is not the only area of the public sector which is facing such changes. The NHS is the area which has been most noticeably addressed. For example, the planned introduction of private prisons has not excited widespread public concern.

12

Drawing the Threads Together

Nurses, together with their patients, are suffering from the present economic policies for the Health Service. In particular, there are endless complaints about understaffing. It affects everything that nurses do. Too much work is being done by too few nurses. The quality of nursing care does seem to be falling. It is not surprising that nurses are leaving or thinking of leaving. It is surprising that more nurses have not left. Because their patients need them and because many feel they have a vocation, nurses stay. How much abuse of nurses' goodwill is needed before there is a mass exodus from the Health Service? Already shortages are being experienced in metropolitan areas and especially in London. Too few nurses are being recruited. Too few people, in other words, are interested in nursing. The bad news of the conditions under which nurses have to work has spread. Nursing as an occupation, let alone a career, would receive few whole-hearted recommendations from nurses. Lack of alternative employment may ensure that some recruits are found. However, the inability of the Health Service to attract sufficient recruits to nursing surely reflects the recent treatment of nurses in the NHS. After all, the much-heralded demographic time bomb had not yet arrived.

The failure of the NHS to meet the demands of its nursing workforce is in part due to the fact that most are women. Pay levels, lack of training opportunities, promotion, childcare, and flexible hours, all reveal a perception of a workforce which is easily replaced. Such a workforce exerts little pressure for change. It is 17 years since the Briggs Committee reported. Many of the problems they identified are not only still present but have worsened. This is, in part, due to a limited view of women and their jobs. In this view, women only play at their jobs. Women's work is seen as being of secondary importance to the real business of marriage or bringing up children. Of course if you treat your workforce badly enough marriage and bringing up children can easily be seen as welcome interruptions to an unsatisfying and frustrating career. There is the ring of a self-fulfilling prophecy here.

Nurses do not simply work for money. Self-righteous acceptance by the government of the recommendations of the Pay Review Body in 1988, so much heralded by the media, illustrates the dominant and blinkered view of why nurses work. Adequate pay, is a necessary but not a sufficient condition for retaining a nursing workforce. Nurses have many demands as employees and as women which are not being met.

In addressing the 'problem' of nurses leaving the NHS a number of influential, and not always obvious, factors have been uncovered. Firstly, that nurses are seen as a *disposable workforce*, use-once-and-throw-away, emerges in a number of different contexts. There is a failure to develop nurses and to maximize their potential, at all levels in nursing. Learners do not seem to be treated as a valuable workforce. Support for the learners as they go through their baptism by fire comes from their peers rather than from 'the system'. Evidence that nurses are seen as a disposable workforce can also be found in the increasing amount of work they have to do. Understaffing is the most prominent complaint from these nurses. There is no 'slack' to be found in nurses' work. There is little or no time to sit and chat with the patients or even to do the little tasks which make the patients' lives more tolerable. Rushing around doing the bare essentials ensures that as standards fall, so does morale. Managers and administrators making precise calculations as to how many nurses are required for *x* number of patients, ignore the needs of patients as people. Nursing is becoming, at least in the NHS, task-centred rather than people-centred. However, as the nurses have attested, the pleasure they obtain from nursing comes not from the tasks themselves but from the people – their patients. But the interests of nurses are not being taken into account at the moment. Too great a concern with statistics has displaced attention from any concern with retaining a skilled workforce. The economic stringencies currently being imposed on the NHS are strengthening the view of nurses as being a disposable workforce.

The dominant priority within the NHS is towards cure rather than care. In pursuing this priority most emphasis is given to the benefits of a steadily increasing through-put of patients. Quantity is the watchword, while quality can easily be overlooked when it does not appear in the accountants' reports. The dominance of cure over care also means that the expressive skills of nurses are downgraded in importance. In this view good nurses are specialist, technically orientated nurses. Yet it is a view which contrasts vividly with that of nurses themselves. For nurses themselves, the 'good nurse' is caring, thoughtful, and compassionate. The good nurse is aware of the needs of the patient. Very seldom do nurses make the link between being a good nurse and a skilled nurse. The emphasis in *Project 2000* on the 'specialist practitioner' and the 'knowledgeable doer' seems to have little to do with the priorities of nurses.

The search for professional status by some nurses can be interpreted as a rebuttal of the importance of the expressive skills long associated with nursing. Such skills have a restricted place in the 'scientific' view of health care. Does the implementation of the recommendations of *Project 2000* mean that a redefinition of nursing, in line with the priorities of the medical profession, has been effected? Quite clearly many of the nurses I spoke to are anti-academic. There is likely to be a clash of perspectives when the first batch of nurses trained in polytechnics enter the ranks of nurses. The originators of the recommendations in *Project 2000* have their own view of nursing. In some respects, it is a view which finds little echo amongst the nurses I talked to. Nurses see themselves as practical people rather than theoretical.

There *is* common agreement that learners should be supernumerary. Everyone is aware that learners' training needs are given insufficient attention. Learners, in being treated simply as a pair of hands, suffer from being part of a disposable workforce. For *Project 2000* to be successful, the increasingly expensive nursing workforce will have to be carefully nurtured. And, as nurses become scarce, they will find their conditions of employment improve. But at the same time there will need to be a change of attitude amongst senior managers and administrators in the Health Service towards nurses and women.

Not surprisingly *gender* is an extremely important factor in explaining the situation of nurses. Gender is influential from two perspectives. Firstly, from the perspective of managers and administrators who see women as somehow only playing, and temporarily, at a job. Thus, for example, there is little point in making any great investment in the training of women, or in seeking to provide them with career and promotion opportunities. As they have been easily replaceable why bother to mess about with childcare facilities and flexible hours of working?

Gender is also influential, perhaps even more so, in the perspectives of nurses themselves. In some respects, nurses are *their own worst enemies*. Many nurses seem to collude in maintaining the traditional subservient attitude towards the medical profession. In adopting anti-academic attitudes, nurses accentuate the difference between doctors and nurses. Thus nurses can be viewed as limited in potential by members of the medical profession. At the same time nurses come to see themselves as not as good as the medical profession. Nurses frequently complain about the bitchiness in nursing. On analysis it emerges that nurses do not appear to sufficiently value the work and the skills of their nursing colleagues. Nurses are unsympathetic to their colleagues. Colleagues are not given the support they need and want. Are the attitudes of nurses towards one another merely reflecting the misogynistic attitudes sometimes found in the ranks of the medical profession? Perhaps the anti-academic sentiments are used as a justification by nurses in order to accept their own subservient position? It is predictable, given the way that nurses are treated as employees, that nurses' perception of one another is negative. Negative reinforcement is also given through the attitudes and behaviour of some members of the medical profession towards nurses. In contrast, patients see nurses positively. It is reasonable, therefore, that nurses' job satisfaction should come from patients.

Potentially nurses could gain other satisfactions from their work such as respect of nursing colleagues and those in the medical profession. That such respect is seldom on offer now may be due to the present system of nurse training. Once nurse training is removed to polytechnics and colleges the influence of the, often conservative, traditions within nursing may be diminished. Similarly the degree of deference given to members of the medical profession may be reduced when nurses become part of the world of higher education. The presently closed and self-reinforcing system of nurse training is long overdue for change. Nevertheless, the repercussions of implementing the planned changes will be substantial. Divisions will be created between the 'old brigade' and the new. Change will, as ever, be resisted. Not only by nurses but by others in the health-care team. In a search for a new identity nursing will come up against entrenched vested interests. In particular the stance adopted by the medical profession to the changes in nurse education will be crucial. If the medical profession continues to withhold due respect from nurses, then *Project 2000* may well encounter obstacles.

It is not clear how successful *Project 2000* can be. Many of the difficulties identified in nursing are likely to obstruct any real changes in nursing. Nursing is hierarchical, often conservative and there is a dislike of those who 'speak out'. The ethos of 'not rocking the boat' ensures that poor nursing practices are not addressed; reasonable complaints cannot be made and suggestions for change are received in silence. Issues which ought to have been confronted go unchallenged. *Project 2000* may simply be skirting round some of these fundamental difficulties in nursing.

Of course, *Project 2000* may, by tackling some issues, cause changes to be effected elsewhere. For example, by removing nurse training from the practical setting to the academic setting may act to weaken the sense of vocation to be found amongst nurses. Although it is envisaged that learners will still have substantial experience in a practical setting, their initial point of reference may be the polytechnic rather than the NHS. Nursing may become just another qualification rather than a special one involving a sense of dedication. In turn, given the greater association with trainees in other fields, nurse learners will develop a greater degree of self-worth particularly with respect to pay. The promotion and career opportunities offered to nurses will also have to improve. But it should not be forgotten that these changes, exciting in prospect though they may be, are for the minority of those involved in caring.

The removal of the enrolled nurse grade, the relatively small amount of training given to the new grade of 'helper' will act to deskill the jobs of many women. For those who are unwilling or unable to meet the qualifications for registered nurse training, the alternative is a job with less training and, inevitably, less pay and prospects. These women, and they will be women, will be paying for the low-cost solutions being found to meet the rising costs of health care.

Other women will be paying for another low-cost solution: the increasing emphasis on care in the community. The euphemism of 'community' misleads. People who were previously patients in mental hospitals will be looked after by members of their families, usually women. Hidden in private houses, these ex-patients and their suffering relatives will be out of sight and out of mind, saving the government money all the while. It must not be forgotten that many of the problems being faced by nurses, patients, and the NHS are problems which have been created by deliberate political and economic policies.

By listening to nurses talking about their work the relationships between the individual and the political have become clearer. Through their accounts of nursing, the effects of ever-tightening budgets are made real. In emphasizing the individuals' accounts and identifying areas of difficulty, it is too easy to blame individuals and to lose sight of the basic constraints on their actions. The world of nurses is simply a reflection of the wider society. But that does not mean it cannot be changed.

Appendices

APPENDIX 1: *Notes on the research and methodology*

The research on which this book is based started in 1985. At that time the University of Lancaster was approached by a District Health Authority which wishes to remain anonymous, to investigate 'the problem' of nurse wastage. It was felt that too many nurses were leaving the Health Authority. In order to gain an appreciation of the issues involved a pilot study was undertaken in late 1985 by Dr John Hockey (findings from this pilot study were published, see Hockey, J. (1987) 'A Picture of Pressure', *Nursing Times*, 8th July, 83:27).

Following on from this initial survey, a fully-fledged investigation into issues surrounding nurse recruitment and wastage was mounted. It was funded by the Leverhulme Trust and began in April 1986. The project lasted for 2 years and received the full co-operation of the Health Authority to whom our thanks must go. Throughout the research the Health Authority has continued to give every assistance to the research team for which we are most appreciative and grateful.

The views and opinions were obtained of over 700 nurses working in a variety of settings in one Health Authority. It is in a region which gained from the re-allocation of resources within the NHS. The policy of re-allocating resources aimed to ensure a fairer distribution of resources within the NHS (see DHSS 1976; separate Reports on resource allocation were produced in Scotland, Wales, and Northern Ireland). The policy meant that some areas which had traditionally enjoyed extensive health care facilities were given fewer resources. Regions which had traditionally been less well endowed with health care facilities were given greater resources. Thus, the area in which the research took place was facing better general conditions than many others in England and Wales. It is an area in which there is, as yet, no great shortage of nurses and in that respect it differs from some metropolitan areas in the UK. Hence, we were not in an area where particular difficulties would be expected. It is, therefore, a good area on which to test the general situation regarding nursing. The terms and conditions of employment for nurses in this Health Authority are not substantially different from those elsewhere in Britain. So while the nurses who were interviewed or completed a questionnaire are not a representative sample of nurses throughout Britain, I suspect that the experiences they report and the comments they make will find echoes amongst their colleagues elsewhere. In short, I do not think their accounts of nursing are likely to differ greatly from those of other nurses working in the NHS.

The information we obtained came from five sources: (a) A questionnaire survey which produced 589 completed questionnaires. One hundred and fifty-four questionnaires came from nurses who had left the employment of the Health Authority in the preceding 15 months; and 435 came from nurses who remained in the employment of the Health Authority. (A 'Sourcebook' giving the detailed findings from the questionnaire has been produced by Paul Bagguley: (1988) *A Report of a Study of Turnover and Work Dissatisfaction amongst UK Professional Nurses*, University of Lancaster, Department of Sociology.) A pilot survey for the questionnaire was conducted amongst nurses working in another Health Authority in the same region. (b) One hundred nurses were interviewed: fifty were nurses who left during the months of November 1986–January 1987 and fifty were nurses employed by the Health Authority. (c) A cohort of ten pupil nurses and a cohort of eleven student nurses undertaking general nurse training were interviewed at intervals during their first year. (d) Seven nursing officers were interviewed. (e) Finally, as the research was being carried out, informal conversations and observations were taking place all the time. Such sources of information are important: chance comments lead to new perspectives and redefinitions of the research.

For the most part, earlier researchers (see Appendix 2) had concentrated solely on the collection of quantitative data to find out why nurses were leaving the NHS (two studies, L. Hockey (1976) in Scotland and the DHSS (1972), did collect quantitative data). Our aim was to find out what lay behind the statistics. Statistics can be useful as benchmarks and indicators of underlying problems. They seldom, on their own, reveal the depth and breadth of experiences. In such research, nurses' own accounts of their situation are often neglected. As a point of departure, we carried out our own questionnaire survey amongst the nurses who were employed by, or who had recently left the employment of, the Health Authority. However, the main emphasis and my main interest was in the interview survey of nurses and learners. It is on these that this book is principally based. There are references to the questionnaire findings, but for the most part the nurses who were interviewed are the focus of attention.

For ease of presentation the nurses who left the Health Authority are referred to as 'leavers' and those who remained in the Health Authority as 'stayers'. However, it must be stressed that these 'leavers' may be temporary or permanent leavers. For example, one nurse could have been taking maternity leave while another was going abroad to nurse. The first may intend to return to the NHS while the latter may never even return to the UK. Similarly, today's 'stayers' may well be yesterday's or tomorrow's 'leavers'. The categories are, in that sense, artificial and that should be borne in mind.

The nurses came from all areas of health care ranging from mental handicap, general nursing, midwifery, mental illness as well as from the community and from all grades from enrolled nurses up to and including sister/charge nurse level. Learners were included but nursing assistants and auxiliaries were excluded. A small number of nursing officers were also included in the interview sample (for details of the samples obtained see Appendices 3–5).

APPENDIX 2: *Previous research: a brief overview*

A good deal of research concerned with nurses and nurse learners has been undertaken in the fairly recent past. The focus of attention varied. For example, Birch, investigated why nurse learners left during training (Birch, J. (1975) *To Nurse or Not to Nurse: An Investigation into the Causes of Withdrawal During Nurse Training*, London, Royal College of Nursing). In 1976, Lisbeth Hockey reported on a survey of nurses in Scotland which looked at wider issues related to women (Hockey, L. (1976) *Women in Nursing*, London, Hodder & Stoughton). Mercer reported in 1979 on labour turnover amongst nurses (Mercer, G.M. (1979) *The Employment of Nurses*, London, Croom Helm). Moores *et al.* in 1982 conducted research into the attitudes of nurses to aspects of their work (Moores, B. *et al.* (1982) 'Attitudes of 2325 active and inactive nurses to aspects of their work', *Journal of Advanced Nursing*, 7, 483–9 and Moores, B. *et al.* (1983) 'An analysis of the factors which impinge on a nurse's decision to enter, stay in, leave or re-enter the nursing profession', *Journal of Advanced Nursing*, 8, 227–35. In the immediate past, the Confederation of Health Service Employees (COHSE) has conducted a survey of nurses' opinions on various topics which was presented in evidence to the Pay Review Body for Nurses and Midwives in 1986 (Confederation of Health Service Employees (1987) *Nurses and Midwives' Survey*, Banstead, COHSE – unpublished). Also, the Institute of Manpower Studies has completed research for the Royal College of Nursing (RCN) into the supply and demand for nurses (Waite, R. and Hutt, R. (1987) *Attitudes, Jobs and Mobility of Qualified Nurses: a report for the Royal College of Nursing*, Brighton, Institute of Manpower Studies, Report No. 130 (the sample was restricted to members of the Royal College of Nursing). Some interesting research into recruitment and wastage has also been undertaken in Ireland under the direction of Andrew Young (Young, A. (1983) *Factors Affecting the Recruitment and Wastage of Nurses in Northern Ireland*, New University of Ulster, unpublished; Department of Health and Social Security (1984) *Nursing in the 80's*, Belfast, DHSS. For a review of the literature on absence and wastage amongst trained nurses prior to 1978, see Redfern, S.J. (1978) 'Absence and wastage in trained nurses: a selective review of the literature', *Journal of Advanced Nursing*, 3, 231–49.

In an excellent piece of work, a comprehensive statement about the conditions and experiences of nurses at the beginning of the 1970s was made by the Briggs Committee which reported in 1972 (Department of Health and Social Security (1972) *Report of the Committee on Nursing*, London, HMSO, Cmnd 5115 (The Briggs Report)).

APPENDIX 3: *Questionnaire sample composition*

	Stayers		Leavers		Combined	
	No.	%	No.	%	No.	%
Grade						
Sister	99	22.8	15	9.7	114	19.3
Staff nurse	145	33.3	60	39.0	205	34.8
Enrolled nurse	116	26.7	27	17.5	143	24.3
Learners	75	17.2	52	33.8	127	21.6
Total	435	100.0	154	100.0	589	100.0
Age						
Under 20	7	1.6	—	—	7	1.2
20–24	106	24.4	60	39.0	166	28.2
25–29	97	22.3	32	20.8	129	21.9
30–34	62	14.2	22	14.3	84	14.3
35–39	61	14.0	13	8.4	74	12.6
40–44	42	9.7	11	7.1	53	9.0
45–49	21	4.8	3	1.9	24	4.1
50–54	26	6.0	4	2.6	30	5.1
Over 55	13	3.0	9	5.8	22	3.7
Total	435	100.0	154	99.9	589	100.1
Gender						
Female	389	89.4	140	90.9	529	89.8
Male	46	10.6	14	9.1	60	10.2
Total	435	100.0	154	100.0	589	100.0
Location						
General hospital	212	48.7	63	40.9	275	46.7
Community service	35	8.0	12	7.8	47	8.0
Midwifery	61	14.0	20	13.0	81	13.7
Psychiatric	61	14.0	14	9.1	75	12.7
Mental Handicap	3	.7	—	—	3	.5
School of Nursing	63	14.5	45	29.2	108	18.3
Total	435	99.9	154	100.0	589	99.9
Marital status						
Single	142	32.6	73	47.4	215	36.5
Married	293	67.4	79	52.3	372	63.2
Missing	—	—	2	2.3	2	.3
Total	435	100.0	154	102.0	589	100.0

APPENDIX 4: *Interview sample composition*

	Stayers		Leavers		Total	
	No.	%	No.	%	No.	%
Grade						
Sister/Charge N.	14	28.0	13	26.0	27	27.0
Staff nurse	16	32.0	19	38.0	35	35.0
Enrolled nurse	12	24.0	15	30.0	27	27.0
Learners	8	16.0	3	6.0	11	11.0
Total	50	100.0	50	100.0	100	100.0
Age						
Under 20	1	2.0	—	—	1	1.0
20–24	10	20.0	12	24.0	22	22.0
25–29	14	28.0	16	32.0	30	30.0
30–34	6	12.0	8	16.0	14	14.0
35–39	7	14.0	10	20.0	17	17.0
40–44	3	6.0	—	—	3	3.0
45–49	3	6.0	2	4.0	5	5.0
50–54	3	6.0	1	2.0	4	4.0
Over 55	3	6.0	1	2.0	4	4.0
Total	50	100.0	50	100.0	100	100.0
Gender						
Female	45	90.0	45	90.0	90	90.0
Male	5	10.0	5	10.0	10	10.0
Total	50	100.0	50	100.0	100	100.0
Location						
General hospital	27	54.0	29	58.0	56	56.0
Community service	3	6.0	3	6.0	6	6.0
Midwifery	2	4.0	6	12.0	8	8.0
Psychiatric	9	18.0	8	16.0	17	17.0
Mental Handicap	1	2.0	1	2.0	2	2.0
School of Nursing	8	16.0	3	6.0	11	11.0
Total	50	100.0	50	100.0	100	100.0
Number of years in nursing:						
1–4 years	13	26.0	9	18.0	22	22.0
5–9 years	16	32.0	20	40.0	36	36.0
10–14 years	10	20.0	18	36.0	28	28.0
15–19 years	4	8.0	—	—	4	4.0
Over 20 years	7	14.0	3	6.0	10	10.0
Total	50	100.0	50	100.0	100	100.0

APPENDIX 4 (*cont.*)

	Stayers		Leavers		Total	
	No.	%	No.	%	No.	%
Marital status:						
Single	22	44.0	18	36.0	40	40.0
Married	28	56.0	32	64.0	60	60.0
Total	50	100.0	50	100.0	100	100.0

APPENDIX 5: *Learners' sample composition*

	Pupils		Students		All learners	
Age	No.	%	No.	%	No.	%
Under 20	5	50.0	6	54.5	11	52.4
20–24	4	40.0	3	27.3	7	33.3
25–29	1	10.0	1	9.1	2	9.5
30–34	—	—	1	9.1	1	4.8
Total	10	100.0	11	100.0	21	100.0

There was only one male learner: a student nurse.

Marital status						
Married/partner	2	20.0	2	18.2	4	19.0
Single	8	80.0	9	81.8	17	81.0
Total	10	100.0	11	100.0	21	100.0

APPENDIX 6: *Number of children*

	Stayers		Leavers		Total	
	No.	%	No.	%	No.	%
Questionnaire respondents						
One	74	17.0	24	15.6	98	16.6
Two	95	21.8	15	9.7	110	18.7
Three or more	27	6.2	13	8.4	40	6.8
None	239	54.9	102	66.2	341	57.9
Total	435	99.9	154	99.9	589	100.0

APPENDIX 6: (*cont.*)

	Stayers		Leavers		Total	
	No.	%	No.	%	No.	%
Interview respondents						
One	3	6.0	8	16.0	11	11.0
Two	14	28.0	10	20.0	24	24.0
Three or more	7	14.0	7	14.0	14	14.0
None	26	52.0	25	50.0	51	51.0
Total	50	100.0	50	100.0	100	100.0

(Figures; in this and subsequent tables, may not add to 100 due to rounding)

APPENDIX 7: *Number of breaks from nursing*

	Stayers		Leavers		Total	
	No.	%	No.	%	No.	%
One	110	25.3	46	29.9	156	26.5
Two	35	8.0	18	11.7	53	9.0
Three of more	22	5.1	14	9.1	36	6.1
None	252	57.9	69	44.8	321	54.5
Missing	16	3.7	7	4.5	23	3.9
Total	435	100.0	154	100.0	589	100.0

APPENDIX 8: *Why returned to nursing*
Questionnaire respondents only:
'If you have had breaks, what made you decide to return to NHS nursing?'

	Stayers		Leavers	
	No.	%	No.	%
Needed the money	108	63.5	26	33.3
Able to leave family	97	57.1	25	32.0
Wanted to get out of house	53	31.2	15	19.2
Preferred NHS working conditions	30	17.6	14	17.9
Family/own health	16	9.4	1	1.3
Preferred NHS nursing pay	10	5.9	6	7.7
	(*n*=170)		(*n*=78)	

(Number of nurses mentioning each aspect)

APPENDIX 9: *Doing other's work*
'In the last week have you done work which ought really to have been done by
each of the type of staff listed below?'
(Asked in stayers' questionnaire only)

	No.	%
Domestic staff	265	60.6
Clerical staff	241	55.1
Messengers	201	46.0
Less highly qualified nurses than you	167	38.2
More highly qualified nurses than you	148	33.9
Doctors	139	31.8
Social workers	95	21.7
Other professional or technical staff	79	18.1
None of these	45	10.3

APPENDIX 10: *Community care*
'How do you feel about the present moves to community care?'

	Stayers		Leavers			Total
	No.	%	No.	%	No.	%
Approve/strongly	232	53.3	92	59.7	324	55.0
Disapprove/strongly	60	13.8	14	9.1	74	12.6
Unsure/indifferent	143	32.9	48	31.2	191	32.4
Total	435	100.0	154	100.0	589	100.0

Bibliography

Abel-Smith, B. (1960) *A History of the Nursing Profession*, London, Heinemann.

Abel-Smith, B. (1976) *Value for money in Health Services*, London, Heinemann.

Abel-Smith, B. (1978) *The National Health Service: the first thirty years*, London, HMSO.

Ackroyd, S. (1987) *Report of the Exploratory Study of Morale Amongst Nurses in the Acute Unit of Lancaster District Health Authority*, University of Lancaster, Department of Behaviour in Organizations – unpublished.

Alleway, L. (1987) 'Make or break?', *Nursing Times*, 6 May, 83:18, 25–6.

Altschul, A.T. (1979) 'Commitment to nursing', *Journal of Advanced Nursing*, 4:2, 123–5.

Altschul, A.T. (1983) 'With all due respect . . .', *Nursing Mirror*, 13 July, 157:2, 20.

Anderson, G. and Barnett, J. (1986) 'Nurse appraisal in practice', *The Health Service Journal*, 30 October, 96:5023, 1420–1.

Anderson, O. (1987) 'A national health service – in reality what can that mean?', *The Health Service Journal*, 29 January, 98:5035, 126–8.

Annandale-Steiner, D. (1979) 'Unhappiness is the nurse who expected more', *Nursing Mirror*, 29 November, 34–6.

Ashley, J.A. (1980) 'Power in structured misogyny', *Advances in Nursing Science*, 2:3, 3.

Austin, J.K., Champion, V.L. and Tzeng, O.C.S. (1985) 'Crosscultural comparison on nursing image', *International Journal of Nursing Studies*, 22:3, 231–9.

Bagguley, P. (1988) *A Report of a Study of Turnover and Work Dissatisfaction amongst UK Professional Nurses*, University of Lancaster, Department of Sociology.

Batchelor, I. (1984) 'Contrast between the professions' in Duncan, A. and McLachlan, G. (eds) *Hospital Medicine and Nursing in the 1980s: Interaction Between the Professions of Medicine and Nursing*, London, Nuffield Provincial Hospitals Trust.

Bell, C. and Roberts, H. (eds) (1984) *Social Researching: Politics, Problems, Practice*, London, RKP.

Birch, J. (1975) *To Nurse or Not to Nurse: An Investigation into the Causes of Withdrawal During Nurse Training*, London, Royal College of Nursing.

Birch J. (1979) 'The anxious learners', *Nursing Mirror*, 7 February 148:6, 17–22.

Blair, P. (1984) 'Why the waste?', *Nursing Focus*, January, 4.

Bond, J. and Bond, S. (1980) 'Sociology: in touch with reality', *Nursing Mirror*, 28 February, 150:9, 27–30.

Bosanquet, N. (1985) 'Where have all the nurses gone?', *Nursing Times*, 23 October, 16–17.

Bosanquet, N. and Gerard, K. (1985) *Nursing Manpower: Recent Trends and Policy Options*, University of York, Centre for Health Economics, Discussion Paper 9.

Bradshaw, P.L. (1984) 'A quaint philosophy', *Senior Nurse*, 28 November, 1:35, 11.

Bradshaw, P. (1986) 'Think before we link', *Nursing Times*, 9 April, 82:15, 51–2.

Braito, R. and Caston, R. (1983) 'Factors influencing job satisfaction in nursing practice' *in* Chaska, N. (ed.) *The Nursing Profession: a Time to Speak*, New York, McGraw Hill.

Brindle, D. (1988a) 'RCN keeps no-strike line', *The Guardian*, 29 March.

Brindle, D. (1988b) 'Pay and privilege on trial', *The Guardian*, 18 May.

Brooks, F., Long, A. and Rathwell, T. (1987) *Midwives' Perceptions of the State of Midwifery*, University of Leeds, Nuffield Centre for Health Services Studios.

Brown A. (1981) 'Going, going . . . gone?', *Nursing Mirror*, 2 April, 152:14, 8.

Brown, R.G.S. and Stones, R.W.H. (1973) *The Male Nurse*, London, G. Bell.

Brunning, H. and Huffington, C. (1985) 'Altered images', *Nursing Times*, 31 July, 81:31, 24–7.

Buchan, J. (1987) 'A shared future', *Nursing Times*, 28 January, 83:4, 44–5.

Cain, A. (1985) 'Constructive criticism', *Nursing Mirror*, 30 October, 161:18, 55–8.

Carpenter, M. (1978) 'Managerialism and the division of labour in nursing', *in* Dingwall, R. and McIntosh, J. (eds) *Readings in the Sociology of Nursing*, Edinburgh, Churchill Livingstone.

Carpenter, M. (1982) 'The labour movement in the National Health Service (NHS): UK', *in* Sethi, A.S. and Dimmock, S.J. (eds) *Industrial Relations and Health Services*, London, Croom Helm.

Castledine, G. (1983) 'Opening the gates on gender traits', *Nursing Mirror*, 13 April, 156:15, 16.

Chapman, C.M. (1977) 'Image of the nurse', *International Nursing Review*, 24, 166–70.

Chapman, C. (1979) 'Sociological theory related to nursing' *in* Colledge, M. and Jones, D. (eds) *Readings in Nursing*, Edinburgh, Churchill Livingstone.

Cherniss, C. (1980) *Professional Burnout in Human Service Occupations*, New York, Praeger.

Clark, J. (1975) *Time Out? A Study of Absenteeism Among Nurses*, London, Royal College of Nursing.

Clark, J. (1979) 'The British National Health Service 1948–1978; should we start again?', *Journal of Advanced Nursing*, 4:2, 205–14.

Clark, J.M. and Redfern, S.J. (1978) 'Absence and wastage in nursing', *Nursing Times*, 20 April, 74:11 (occasional paper), 41–4.

Clark, M.O. (1984) *in* Duncan, A. and McLachlan, G. (eds) *Hospital Medicine and Nursing in the 1980s: Interaction Between the Professions of Medicine and Nursing*, London, Nuffield Provincial Hospitals Trust.

Clarke, M. (1978) 'Getting through the work' *in* Dingwall, R. and McIntosh, J. (eds) *Readings in the Sociology of Nursing*, Edinburgh, Churchill Livingstone.

Cochrane, A.L. (1972) *Effectiveness and Efficiency: Random Reflections on the Health Service*, London, The Nuffield Provincial Hospitals Trust.

Cole, A. (1987) 'On the move', *Nursing Times*, 13 May, 83:19, 16, 18–19.

Colledge, M. and Jones, D. (eds) (1979) *Readings in Nursing*, Edinburgh, Churchill Livingstone.

Confederation of Health Service Employees (1985) *Nurses and Midwives Survey*, Banstead, COHSE – unpublished.

Conway, M.E. (1983) 'Socialization and roles in nursing', *Annual Review of Nursing Research*, 1, 183–208.

Cousins, C. (1987) *Controlling Social Welfare: A Sociology of State Welfare, Work and Organisation*, Brighton, Wheatsheaf.

Cox, D. (1986) *Implementing Griffiths at District Level: report on work in progress*, Paper given to BSA Medical Sociology Conference – unpublished.

Cumberlege, J. (1986) *Neighbourhood Nursing – a Focus for Care*, London, HMSO.

Daniel, W.W. (1969) 'Industrial behaviour and orientation to work – a critique', *Journal of Management Studies*, 6, 366–75.

Darbyshire, P. (1987) 'The burden of history', *Nursing Times*, 28 January, 83:4, 32–4.

Davidson, N. (1987) *A Question of Care: the Changing Face of the National Health Service*, London, Michael Joseph.

Davies, C. (1986) 'Nurse odyssey 2000', *The Health Service Journal*, 24 July, 96:5009, 986–7.

Dean, D.J. (1974) 'Severalls Hospital' *in* Revans, R. (ed.) *Hospital Communication – Choice and Change*, London, Tavistock.

De La Cuesta, C. (1983) 'The nursing process: from development to implementation' *Journal of Advanced Nursing*, 8, p. 365–71.

Department of Health and Social Security (undated) *The Senior Nursing Organisation in Hospitals: An Introduction to the Report of the Salmon Committee*, London, HMSO.

Department of Health and Social Security (undated) *Nursing in the 80's*, Belfast, DHSS.

Department of Health and Social Security (1972) *Report of the Committee on Nursing*, London, HMSO, Cmnd. 5115 (The Briggs Committee).

Department of Health and Social Security (1976) *Sharing Resources for Health in England*, Report of the Resources Allocation Working Party, London, HMSO.

Department of Health and Social Security (1979) *Patients First*, London, HMSO.

Department of Health and Social Security (1982) *Nurse Manpower: Maintaining the Balance*, London, HMSO.

Department of Health and Social Security (1986a) *Fourth Report of the Social Services Committee 1985–6*, London, HMSO.

Department of Health and Social Security (1986b) *Control of Nursing*

Manpower (Fourteenth Report from the Committee of Public Accounts Session 1985–6), London, HMSO.

Devlin, B. (1987) 'An unreal brave new world?', *Nursing Times*, 6 May, 83:18, 29–30.

Dewe, P.J. (1987) 'Identifying strategies nurses use to cope with work stress', *Journal of Advanced Nursing*, 12:4, 489–97.

Dex, S. (1984) *Women's work histories: an Analysis of the Women and Employment Survey*, London, Department of Employment, Research Paper Number 46.

Dex, S. (1985) *The Sexual Division of Work*, Brighton, Harvest Press.

Dex, S. (1987) *Women's Occupational Mobility: a Lifetime Perspective*, London, Macmillan.

Dickson, N. (1986) 'The Future with Confidence', *Nursing Times*, 5 November, 82:45, 50–1.

Dickson, N. (1987) 'Best foot forward', *Nursing Times*, 7 January, 83:1, 40–1.

Dimmock, S. (1986) 'Machiavellian machinations', *Nursing Times*, 9 April, 82:15, 35–6.

Dingwall, R. (1978) 'Getting through the work' *in* Dingwall, R. and McIntosh, J. (eds) *Readings in the Sociology of Nursing*, Edinburgh, Churchill Livingstone.

Dingwall, R. (1979) 'The place of men in nursing' *in* Colledge, M. and Jones, D. (eds) *A Reader in Nursing*, Edinburgh, Churchill Livingstone.

Dingwall, R. and McIntosh, J. (eds) (1978) *Readings in the Sociology of Nursing*, Edinburgh, Churchill Livingstone.

Dolan, N. (1987) 'The relationship between burnout and job satisfaction in nurses', *Journal of Advanced Nursing*, 12:1, 3–12.

Draper, P., Grenholm, G. and Best, G. (1976) *in* Tuckett (ed.) *An Introduction to Medical Sociology*, London, Tavistock.

Duncan, A. and McLachlan, G. (eds) (1984) *Hospital Medicine and Nursing in the 1980s: Interaction Between the Professions of Medicine and Nursing*, London, Nuffield Provincial Hospitals Trust.

Duncan, K.D., Gruneberg, M.M. and Wallis, D. (eds) (1980) *Changes in Working Life*, London, Wiley.

Ehrenreich, B. and English, D. (1973) *Witches, Midwives and Nurses: A History of Women Healers*, New York, Feminist Press.

Etzioni, A. (ed.) (1969) *The Semi-Professions and Their Organization*, New York, Free Press.

Ferriman, A. and Wolmar, C. (1986) 'A tale of two systems', *The Observer*, 18 May, 9.

Field, D. (1984) '"We didn't want him to die on his own" – nurses' accounts of nursing dying patients', *Journal of Advanced Nursing*, 9, 59–70.

Finch, J. (1984) '"It's great to have someone to talk to": the ethics and politics of interviewing women', *in* Bell, C. and Roberts, H. (eds) *Social Researching: Politics, Problems, Practice*, London, RKP.

Firth, H. McIntee, J., KcKeown, P. and Britton, P. (1986) 'Interpersonal support amongst nurses', *Journal of Advanced Nursing*, 11:3, 273–82.

Garner, L. (1979) *The NHS: Your Money or Your Life*, Harmondsworth, Penguin.

Gaze, H. (1987) 'Man Appeal', *Nursing Times*, 20 May, 83:20, 24–7.

George, T.B. (1982) 'Development of the self-concept of nurse in nursing students', *Research in Nursing and Health*, 5:4, 191–7.

Gibberd, F.B. (1983) 'The nursing career structure as seen by a hospital doctor', *British Medical Journal*, 12 March, 286: 6368, 913–4.

Glaser, B.G. and Strauss, A.L. (1968) *The Discovery of Grounded Theory*, London, Weidenfeld & Nicolson.

Goldthorpe, J., Lockwood, O., Bechhofer, F. and Platt, J. (1968) *The Affluent Worker: Industrial Attitudes and Behaviour*, Cambridge, CUP.

Greenborough, J.H. (1985) *Second Report on Nursing Staff, Midwives and Health Visitors 1985* (Review Body for Nursing Staff, Midwives, Health Visitors and Professions Allied to Medicine), London, HMSO, Cmnd. 9529.

Griffiths, E.R. (1983) *NHS Management Inquiry*, London, DHSS.

Griffiths, E.R. (1988) *Community Care: Agenda for Action*, (A Report to the Secretary of State for Social Services), London, HMSO.

Hanson, M. and Patchett, T. (1986) 'When the tap runs dry', *Nursing Times*, 31 December, 82: 52, 26–8.

Hardy, L.K. (1984) 'The emergence of nursing leaders – a case of in-spite of, not because-of', *International Nursing Review*, 31:1, 11–15.

Hardy, L.K. (1987) 'The male model', *Nursing Times*, 27 May, 83:21. 36–8.

Harrison, A. and Gretton, J. (eds) (1984) *Health Care UK 1984: an Economic, Social and Policy Audit*, London, Chartered Institute of Public Finance and Accountancy.

Hawkins, K. (1979) 'Why I'm giving up nursing', *Nursing Mirror*, 22 November, 49:21 10.

Health Service Journal, The (1987) 'Shortages for wrong reasons', *The Health Service Journal*, 27 August, 973.

Henderson, V. (1978) 'The concept of nursing', *Journal of Advanced Nursing*, 3, 113–30.

Heyman, R. (1983) 'A personal construct theory approach to the socialization of nursing trainees in two British general hospitals', *Journal of Advanced Nursing*, 8, 59–67.

Hill, J.M.M. and Trist, E.L. (1962) *Industrial Accidents, Sickness and Other Absences*, London, Tavistock.

Hilldrew, P. (1986) 'Nurses fighting GPs for power', *The Guardian*, 21 July, 4.

Hockey, J. (1987) 'A Picture of Pressure', *Nursing Times*, 8 July, 83, 27.

Hockey, L. (1976) *Women in Nursing*, London, Hodder & Stoughton

Hollingworth, S. (1979) 'A challenge for nurse teaching', *Nursing Times*, 26 July, 75:30 1263.

Hospital and Health Services Review (1986) 'Nurses of the Future', *Hospital and Health Services Review*, September, 82:5, 194–5.

Howie, C. (1987a) 'Back breaking work takes its toll', *The Health Service Journal*, 8 January, 97:5032, 34–5.

Howie, C. (1987b) 'Rocky roll', *Nursing Times*, 20 May, 83:20, 20.

Hudson, B. (1987) 'A quiet revolution – late in coming', *The Health Service Journal*, 9 April, 97:5045, 420–1.

Hughes, D. (1988) 'When nurse knows best: some aspects of nurse/doctor interaction in a casualty department', *Sociology of Health and Illness*, March, 10:1, 1–22.

Hutt, A. (1980) 'Shared learning for shared care: multidisciplinary course at the Middlesex Hospital', *Journal of Advanced Nursing*, 5:4, 389–94.

Hyams, J. (1987) 'Nice nurse: shame about the status', *Company*, July, 82, 84, 133.

Ivancevich, J.M. (1986) 'Life events and hassles as predictors of health symptoms, job performance, and absenteeism', *Journal of Occupational Behaviour*, 7, 39–51.

James, N. (1984) 'A postscript to nursing' *in* Bell, C. and Roberts, H. (eds) *Social Researching: Politics, Problems, Practice*, London, RKP.

Johnson, M. (1986) 'A message for the teacher', *Nursing Times*, 31 December, 82:52, 41–3.

Johnson, M.M. and Martin, H.W. (1958) 'A Sociological Analysis of the Nurse Role, *American Journal of Nursing*, 58:3, 373–7.

Jones, S.L. (1976) 'Socialization vs selection factors as sources of student definitions of the nurse role', *International Journal of Nursing Studies*, 13, 135–8.

Joshi, H. (1984) *Women's Participation in Paid Work: Further Analysis of the Women and Employment Survey*, London, Department of Employment, Research Paper Number 45.

Kalisch, B.J. and Kalisch, P. (1977) 'An analysis of the sources of physician–nurse conflict', *Journal of Nursing Administration*, 7:1, 51–7.

Kalisch, P.A. and Kalisch, B.L. (1986) 'A comparative analysis of nurse and physician characters in the entertainment media', *Journal of Advanced Nursing*, 11:2, 179–95.

Katz, F.E. (1969) 'Nurses' *in* Etzioni, A. (ed.) *The Semi-Professions and Their Organization*, New York, Free Press.

Keddy, B., Jones, M., Jacobs, P., Burton, H. and Rogers, M. (1986) 'The doctor–nurse relationship: an historical perspective', *Journal of Advanced Nursing*, 11:6, 745–53.

Kiger, A.M. (1985) '"Mirror, mirror on the wall . . ." Some reflections on the image', *in* The Nursing Studies Association, *The Politics of Progress*, Proceedings of the 19th Annual Study Day of the Nursing Studies Association, University of Edinburgh, 4 May, 1985.

Kratz, C. (1987) 'Training for a takeover', *Nursing Times*, 27 May, 83:21, 16, 18.

Labour Party, The (1977) *The Right to Health*, London, The Labour Party.

Latham, J.P. (1985) 'Absence from work at the Royal Albert Hospital, Lancaster' (MA Thesis), University of Lancaster.

Lawrence, J.C. (1978) 'Male nurses: a different view', *Imprint*, 25:1, 28–30.

Lee, J.M. (1977) 'Nurse bank scheme', *Nursing Times*, 8 December, 73:49, 1926–7.

Lewis, B. (1980) 'Wastage from nurse training', *Nursing Times*, 13 November, 76:46, 2026–9.

Lindop, E. (1987) 'Factors associated with student and pupil nurse wastage', *Journal of Advanced Nursing*, 12, 751–6.

Logan, W. (1986) 'The Scottish experience (Project 2000)', *Nursing Times*, 27 August, 82:35, 49–50.

Lombardi, T. (1987) 'Under control', *Senior Nurse*, 6:5, 8–9.

Lovell, M.C. (1981) 'Silent but perfect 'partners': medicine's use and abuse of women', *Advances in Nursing Science*, 3:1, 25–40.

MacGuire, J. (1969) *Threshold to Nursing*, London, Bell.

McIntosh, J. and Dingwall, R. (1978) 'Teamwork in theory and practice' *in* Dingwall, R. and McIntosh, J. (eds) *Readings in the Sociology of Nursing*, Edinburgh, Churchill Livingstone.

Mackay, L. and Torrington, D. (1986) 'Training in the UK: down but not out' *Journal of European Industrial Training*, 10, 1, 11–16.

Marshall, J. (1980) 'Stress amongst nurses' *in* Cooper, C.L. and Marshall, J. (eds) *White Collar and Professional Stress*, New York, Wiley.

Martin, L. (1986) 'Future tense', *Nursing Times*, 13 August, 82:33, 48–9.

Maslach, C. (1976) 'Burned-out', *Human Behavior*, 5, 16–22.

Mathieson, A. (1984) 'Wasted opportunities', *Nursing Mirror*, 8 February, 158:61 22–3.

Meates, D. (1971) 'Nursing staff sickness and absenteeism in the Medical and Paediatrics Unit', *Nursing Times*, 16 December, 67:50, 197–200.

Melia, K. (1983) 'Students' Views of Nursing', *Nursing Times*, 18 May, 79:20, 24–7.

Melia, K. (1984) 'Student nurses' construction of occupational socialisation', *Sociology of Health and Illness*, 6:2, 132–51.

Menzies, I. (1970) *The Functioning of Social Systems as a Defence Against Anxiety*, London, Tavistock.

Mercer, G.C. (1979) *The Employment of Nurses*, London, Croom Helm.

Mercer, G. (1980) 'Nurse employment and mobility of trained staff', *Nursing Times*, 27 November, 76:48, 2120–2.

Mercer, G. (1985) 'On the move', *Senior Nurse*, 30 January, 2:4, 6–8.

Mercer, G. and Mould, C. (1976a) *An Investigation into the Level and Character of Labour Turnover Amongst Trained Nurses* (Final Report – Nursing Research Project), University of Leeds, Department of Sociology.

Mercer, G. and Mould, C. (1976b) 'Nurses on the move', *Nursing Times*, 25 March, 72:12, 441–3.

Merrison, A. (1979) *Royal Commission on the National Health Service*, London, HMSO, Cmnd. 7615.

Mitchell, R.G. (1984) *in* Duncan, A. and McLachlan, G. (eds) *Hospital Medicine and Nursing in the 1980s's: Interaction between the Professions of Medicine and Nursing*, London, Nuffield Provincial Hospitals Trust.

Mitchell, T. (1984) 'Is nursing any business of doctors?', *Nursing Times*, 9 May, 80:19, 28–32.

Moores, B., Singh, B.B., and Tun, A. (1982) 'Attitudes of 2325 active and inactive nurses to aspects of their work', *Journal of Advanced Nursing*, 7, 483–9.

Moores, B., Singh, B.B. and Tun, A. (1983) 'An analysis of the factors which impinge on a nurse's decision to enter, stay in, leave or re-enter the nursing profession', *Journal of Advanced Nursing*, 8, 227–35.

Morgan, A.P. and McCann, J.M. (1983) 'Nurse–physician relationships: the ongoing conflict', *Nursing Administration Quarterly*, 7:4, 1–7.

Muir Gray, J.A. (1980) 'Warning: cigarettes may do you good', *Nursing Mirror*, 10 April, 150:15, 21–3.

Murray, M. (1983) 'Role conflict and intention to leave nursing', *Journal of Advanced Nursing*, 8, 29–31.

Nolan, J.W. (1985) 'Work patterns of midlife female nurses', *Nursing Research*, May/June, 30:3, 150–4.

Northcott, N. (1987) 'Thanks for the memory', *Senior Nurse*, 6:5, 28.

Nursing Studies Association (1985) *The Politics of Progress*, Proceedings of the 19th Annual Study Day of the Nursing Studies Association, University of Edinburgh, 4 May, 1985.

Nursing Times (1987) 'Ready for lift-off', *Nursing Times*, 28 January, 83:4, 16–19.

Oakley, A. (1981) 'Interviewing women: a contradiction in terms', *in* Roberts, H. (ed.) *Doing Feminist Research*, London, RKP.

Oakley, A. (1984) 'The importance of being a nurse', *Nursing Times*, 12 December, 80:50, 24–7.

Ogier, M. (1981) A study of the leadership style and verbal interactions of ward sisters and nurse learners' (Ph.D. Thesis), London, Birkbeck College.

Pahl, R.E. (1984) *Divisions of Labour*, Oxford, Blackwell.

Pape, R. (1978) 'Touristry: a type of occupational mobility' *in* Dingwall, R. and McIntosh, J. (eds) *Readings in the Sociology of Nursing*, Edinburgh, Churchill Livingstone.

Peach, L. (1986) 'Manpower and personnel policies: the national perspective', *Hospital and Health Services Review*, September, 82:5, 201–4.

Price, K.M. (1984) 'A study of short-term absence from work among a group of third year student nurses', *Journal of Advanced Nursing*, 9, 493–503.

Promoting Better Health (1987) London, HMSO, Cm.249 (White Paper).

Redfern, S.J. (1978) 'Absence and wastage in trained nurses: a selective review of the literature', *Journal of Advanced Nursing*, 3, 231–49.

Redfern, S.J. (1980) 'Hospital sisters: work attitudes, perceptions and wastage', *Journal of Advanced Nursing*, 5:5, 451–66.

Redfern, S.J. and Spurgeon, P. (1980) 'Job satisfaction and withdrawal of hospital sisters in the UK' *in* Duncan, K.D. *et al. Changes in Working Life*, London, Wiley.

Reid, N.G. (1983) *Nurse Training in the Clinical Area – Volume 1: The Report*, The New University of Ulster.

Reid, N.G. (1985a) 'The effective training of nurses: manpower implications', *International Journal of Nursing Studies*, 22:2, 89–98.

Reid, N.G. (1985b) *Wards in Chancery*, London, Royal College of Nursing.

Revans, R. (1974) *Hospital Communication – Choice and Change*, London, Tavistock.

Roberts, H. (ed.) (1981) *Doing Feminist Research*, London, RKP.

Roberts, K. (1975) 'The developmental theory of occupational choice: a critique and an alternative' *in* Esland, G., Salaman, G., and Speakman, M-A. (eds) *People and Work*, Edinburgh, Holmes McDougall.

Robinson, J. (1986) 'Through the minefield – and into the sun?', *Senior Nurse*, 4:6, 7–9.

Rowden, R. (1984) 'Doctors can work with the nursing process', *Nursing Times*, 9 May, 80:19, 32–4.

Royal College of Nursing (1966) *Comment on Salmon*, London, RCN.

Royal College of Nursing (1978a) *An Assessment of the State of Nursing in the National Health Service*, (RCN submission to the Secretary of State for Social Services), London, RCN.

Royal College of Nursing (1978b) *Counselling*, London, RCN.

Royal College of Nursing (1986) *A Manifesto for Nursing and Health*, London, RCN.

Royal College of Nursing (1987) *Shortage of Nurses in London*, London, RCN.

Royal Commission on the National Health Service (1978) *The Working of the National Health Service*, Research Paper No. 1, London, HMSO.

Rushworth, V. (1975) '"Not in today": absence survey', *Nursing Times*, 11 December, 71:50, 121–4.

Sadler, J. and Whitworth, T. (1975) *Reserves of Nurses*, London, HMSO.

Salvage, J. (1979) 'A crisis of morale?', *Nursing Mirror*, 13 December, 149:24, 14.

Salvage, J. (1985) *The Politics of Nursing*, London, Heinemann.

Salvage, J. and Rogers, R. (1988) *Nurses at Risk: A Guide to Health and Safety at Work*, London, Heinemann.

Schofield, M. (1986) 'Manpower and personnel policies: the district perspective', *Hospital and Health Services Review*, September, 82:5, 204–8.

Scottish Home and Health Department (1975) *The Movements of Hospital Nursing Staff in Scotland*, Edinburgh, Scottish Home and Health Department, Nursing Manpower Planning Report Number 5.

Sethi, A.S. and Dimmock, S. (eds) (1982) *Industrial Relations and Health Services*, London, Croom Helm.

Simpson, R.L. and Simpson, I.H. (1969) 'Women and bureaucracy in the semi-professions', *in* Etzioni, A. (ed.) *The Semi-Professions and Their Organization*, New York, Free Press.

Smith, J.P. (1976) 'Editorial' *Journal of Advanced Nursing*, 1, 339–40.

Smith, M. (1981) 'Nursing Agencies: their value in reducing costs', *Nursing Times*, 26 August, 77:35, 1501–2.

Stannard, C. (1978) 'Old folks and dirty work: the social conditions for patient abuse in a nursing home' *in* Dingwall, R. and McIntosh, J. (eds) *Readings in the Sociology of Nursing*, Edinburgh, Churchill Livingstone.

Stein, L. (1978) 'The doctor-nurse game' *in* Dingwall, R. and McIntosh, J. *Readings in the Sociology of Nursing*, Edinburgh, Churchill Livingstone.

Stewart, B. (1981) 'In need of tender loving care', *Nursing Mirror*, 12 March, 152:11, 35–7.

Stilwell, B. (1986) 'Evolution not revolution', *Senior Nurse*, 4:6, 10–11.

Stoller, E.P. (1978) 'Preconceptions of the Nursing Role: a case study of an entering class', *Journal of Nursing Education*, June, 17:6, 2–14.

Swaffield, L. (1987) 'Ever Ready . . . or Burnt Out?', *Nursing Times*, 25 March 83:12, 25–6.

Taylor, P. (1974) 'Sickness absence: facts and misconceptions', *Journal of the Royal College of Physicians* (London), July, 8:4, 315–33.

Truman, C. (1987) 'Managing the career-break', *Nursing Times*, 21 January, 83:3, 44–5.

Tuckett, D. (ed.) (1976) *An Introduction to Medical Sociology*, London, Tavistock.

Ungerson, C. (1987) *Policy is Personal*, London, Tavistock.

United Kingdom Central Council (1986) *Project 2000*, London, UKCC.

United Kingdom Central Council (1987) *Project 2000: The Final Proposals*, London, UKCC, Project Paper 9.

Waite, R. and Hutt, R. (1987) *Attitudes, Jobs and Moblity of Qualified Nurses: a Report for the Royal College of Nursing*, University of Sussex, Institute of Manpower Studies, IMS Report Number 130.

Walby, S. *Flexibility and the Changing Sexual Division of Labour*, University of Lancaster, Lancaster Regionalism Group, Working Paper 36.

Wandelt, M.A., Pierce, P.M. and Widdowson, R.R. (1981) 'Why nurses leave nursing and what can be done about it' *American Journal of Nursing*, January, 72–7.

Webster, D. (1985) 'Medical students' views of the nurse', *Nursing Research*, 34:5, 313–17.

Weisman, C.S., Alexander, C. and Chase, G. (1981) 'Determinants of hospital staff nurse turnover', *Medical Care*, 19, 431–43.

West, M. and Rushton, R. (1986) The drop-out factor', *Nursing Times*, 31 December, 82:52, 29–31.

Whitehead, M. (1987) *The Health Divide: Inequalities in Health in the 1980's*, London, Health Education Authority.

Whittaker, E. and Olesen, V. (1978) 'The faces of Florence Nightingale: functions of the heroine legend in an occupational sub-culture' *in* Dingwall, R. and McIntosh, J. (eds) *Readings in the Sociology of Nursing*, Edinburgh, Churchill Livingstone.

Wilkinson, R. (1980) How do you stop them leaving?', *Nursing Mirror*, 19 June, 150:19, 43–5.

Wilson-Barnett, J. (1986) 'Ethical dilemmas in nursing', *Journal of Medical Ethics*, 12, 123–6, 135.

World Health Organization (1974) *Community Health Nursing* (Report of a WHO Expert Committee) Geneva, WHO, Technical Report Series Number 558.

World Health Organization (1986) *Having a Baby in Europe*, Geneva, WHO.

Wright, S. (1985) 'New nurses: new boundaries', *Nursing Practice*, 1:1, 32–9.

Young, A. (1983) *Factors Affecting the Recruitment and Wastage of Nurses in Northern Ireland*, New University of Ulster – unpublished.